THE SECRET OF THE SOUL TIE

WHAT THE ENEMY DOES NOT WANT YOU TO KNOW ABOUT UNGODLY AND UNHEALTHY SOUL TIES

JAMES D. EDWARDS

LAKEVIEW
PUBLICATIONS

CONTENTS

PART ONE
THE BIRTHING

I dedicate this book to my 12 year old self. Had I known what I know now, I probably could've avoided a lot of heartbreak, rejection and unnecessary pain.

I dedicate this book to those who have joined themselves knowingly or unknowingly to ungodly or unhealthy attachments. I'm sure you the feel pressure of being entrapped and you have a great desire to experience complete freedom. These truths are specifically for you.

FOREWORD

I am blessed by the accomplishment of James Edwards putting his life to pen and paper, it gives the world an opportunity to see the transforming power of God in the life of someone who was destined to be a negative statistic in the black community and on American itself.

As I read this book the scripture that kept coming to mind is found in Ecclesiastes 4:12 "And if one prevail against him, two shall withstand him; and a threefold cord is not quickly broken."

As you read this book you will be intrigued by the countless stories and life examples that are given. "The Secret of the Soul Tie" causes you to ponder the thought, what am I tied to? I realize that some of us will have to fight through the misinformation that soul ties do not exist while pondering why am I not living in the freedom that God has promised. Reading this book has made me keenly aware that we may have tied ourselves to things that are unprofitable without realizing it. It brings a greater focus to the text found in Hebrews 12:1 "Wherefore seeing we also are compassed about with so great a cloud of witnesses, let us lay aside every weight, and the sin which doth so easily beset us, and let us run with patience the race that is set before us,"

If God could take "Butch" from Alabama, and transform him into "Pastor James" from Texas, if you are willing to let go of those weights and ties that are holding you back, then Jesus can welcome you into His fold and become that 'threefold cord' that is not quickly broken!

Bishop Marvin L. Winans,
Bishop-Elect for Perfecting Fellowship International
Senior Pastor of Perfecting Church
Detroit, MI & Toledo, Ohio

INTRODUCTION

How can I ever forget the morning of May 4, 2021? It was around 10 AM. I was sitting in my office, reading a book, and trying to formulate a thesis or principle for my next sermon. I had just finished morning prayer on Facebook, YouTube, and TikTok, and I was asking God for a sense of direction.

During my reading, I received a notification of a TikTok message from one of my supporters. To be honest, I didn't want to answer it because the trolls are worse in my inbox messenger than when I'm doing a live video. Nevertheless, I opened my TikTok app and read the message.

It was a brother by the name of Kurt, who felt strongly that God was leading him to speak with me, even if it meant he had to pay for a counseling or coaching fee. I sent him the form. He immediately filled it out, and about an hour later, we began our coaching video session.

Kurt introduced himself. He was 39 years old and was looking for spiritual guidance to get his life into a permanent position of peace. While Kurt was sharing his story, he caught my attention as he told me about his last year in college when he was 21 years old. He and his college sweetheart were preparing for their engagement—until he met a woman who was about eight years older than him, at a company where he was interning.

According to Kurt, after about six months into their sexual relationship, she tricked him into breaking up with his college sweetheart. Then he immediately began an exclusive relationship with this woman.

A month after breaking up with his college sweetheart, Kurt moved in with his new girlfriend (and coworker) and began a common-law marriage with her. They were together for about four years when suddenly the unthinkable was revealed. Kurt found out that she was cheating on him with another guy.

Kurt said that he forgave her and tried to reconcile the relationship. Consequently, she refused and moved on with the other guy. Of course, this broke Kurt's heart because he couldn't believe that she would leave him for someone else.

At that point, Kurt was 25 years old. He then tried to get back together with his college sweetheart. To his surprise, Kurt learned that she was deep into a new relationship with another guy. Nevertheless, Kurt met her for lunch one day to apologize for the way he had treated her. He also wanted to show her how much he had changed for the better. She accepted his apology and told him that she was in a relationship with someone else, but if things didn't work out between the two of them, then she would be open to starting over with Kurt.

In Kurt's mind, the door of opportunity was still open, so he remained close by in case things didn't work out between his college sweetheart and her new boyfriend.

Kurt continued telling me his story. After two years of waiting for his college sweetheart, he decided to move on. He entered a relationship with another woman. They were together for five years and had a child together. At this point, his girlfriend wanted to get married, but Kurt wasn't ready. So, the mother of his child moved on because she didn't want to continue playing house with Kurt, without having his last name.

Meanwhile, Kurt's college sweetheart had gotten married. Most of his friends were also married, raising their families, building careers, and accelerating in life. That's when Kurt started feeling the pressure.

At the age of 33, Kurt met his fourth and final girlfriend. They were together for three years and had a child together. This time, Kurt agreed to marry her. According to Kurt, he and his wife were living the typical married life. This is where the story gets interesting.

Kurt said, "Pastor James, I'm 39 years old; I have two kids; my marriage looks great on the outside, but I'm so miserable. I'm dying on the inside. Pastor, I gotta be honest. I am in the marriage, but the marriage isn't in me. I'm not happy. I am always thinking about how my second girlfriend tricked me out of my relationship with my college sweetheart. I think about how she played me, and I always think about how things should've worked out between my first son's mom and me. She wasn't the problem. All she wanted was to make our relation-ship right in the eyes of God, but I was selfish, and Pastor, I just feel trapped in my marriage now. I need help! What's wrong with me? Why am I so messed up like this? How do I change this? Honestly, Pastor, I want to know what you think."

I paused for about five seconds because I wanted to come across as clear, direct, effective, and concise. I took a deep breath and responded. "Kurt, can you handle it real, raw, rugged, and relevant?"

"Yes sir, Pastor! That's exactly why I messaged you, because I knew you were going to keep it 100 with me."

"Kurt, you told me your story, and believe me, I heard every word you said, but more importantly, I heard the spirit behind what you said. Number One, you are struggling with lasciviousness. That means you are wrestling with some uncontrolled lust. You told me about the girlfriends you were committed to in a relationship, but you never told me about the other girls you had sex with in between your committed relationships. I'm 100% sure that in the two years while you were single, you were having sex with other women. Am I right or wrong?"

"You're right, Pastor," Kurt said, a slight smirk on his face.

"That's why I say you're struggling with lasciviousness. Next, it sounds like you have an extreme case of immaturity. I suspect this because you said that your second girlfriend tricked you into leaving your college sweetheart. Listen to me, Kurt. She didn't trick you; you chose to leave. You left because you wanted to leave. And the longer it takes for you to accept the truth within yourself about why you left your college sweetheart, the longer you will stay in bondage to that immaturity. When people refuse to take responsibility for their actions, that's a sign that they are refusing to change their ways.

"And last, it sounds to me as though you're wrestling with some soul ties. You've got a lot of people living inside of you, all at the same time you are married to your wife. In other words, your soul is tied to other souls besides your wife."

"Pastor, you might be right. I might have some strong lust and I might be a little immature, but I don't believe I have any soul ties" Said Kurt.

His response confused me a little. I paused for a second to gather my thoughts. "Why do you think that you don't have any soul ties?"

"Because my pastor said that there is no such thing as a soul tie, and he said that soul ties are not in the Bible."

I was shocked that he rebutted with something his pastor had said. I shifted into apologetic mode, which is a reasoned defense of a belief and doctrine.

"If that's the case, then there is no such thing as the Trinity. If you want to get 100% precise about the wording in the Bible, then I don't see anywhere in the Bible where it uses the word 'Trinity,' but we do know that God is described in the Bible as 'one God who operates and demonstrates three different functions.' He is the Father in creation because in the beginning, God created the Heavens and the Earth [Genesis 1:1]. He's the Son in redemption [Romans 3:24], and He is the Holy Spirit in regeneration [Titus 3:5]. Though I don't see the word 'Trinity' anywhere in the King James Bible, or any other biblical translations, the concept is clearly there. Am I right or wrong?"

"Well, I don't know," Kurt said.

"Oh, but you wanted me to know what your pastor said about soul ties. So apparently you've already been talking to your pastor, and he couldn't help you, but when I give you a new level of truth that you don't want to hear, you deny it. Kurt, I gotta be honest, the best and easiest way for you to stay in bondage is for you to stay in denial."

I continued ministering to Kurt, and as the conversation continued, I heard the Holy Spirit speak to me: *It's time for you to teach a series entitled The Secret of the Soul Tie: What the Enemy Does Not Want You to Know about Ungodly and Unhealthy Soul Ties.*

After the conversation with Kurt was over, I knew exactly what direction God wanted me to go in for that Sunday morning.

THE ENEMY WANTS YOU TO BE IGNORANT

When it comes to controversial topics or taboo subjects—whether biblically or in the church—one principle that life has taught me to live by is this: A man with experience has no business arguing with a man who has only a theory. Kurt came to me for help, but he couldn't receive his breakthrough because he was locked in his own theory. I wasn't offended by his theory. I've been free for over 14 years because I've had a few experiences with ungodly soul ties. Don't get me wrong; this book does not come from one personal experience that doesn't line up with what the Bible teaches. What you will find in this book is information on, a revelation about, and an understanding of the sneaky and deceitful works of demonic oppression regarding ungodly and unhealthy soul ties.

The top three ways the enemy can keep a person in bondage and under demonic oppression are deception, ignorance, and temptation. The word "deception" means "the deliberate act of causing someone to accept something as true or valid, when what they are trying to get them to accept is false and invalid." Night and day Satan is working to trick humankind into becoming an enemy of truth. When a person is an enemy of truth, he or she, unintentionally and unknowingly, becomes an enemy to God.

The Bible says in John 16:13, *"However, when He, the Spirit of Truth, has come, He will guide you into all truth"* (NKJV). What's interesting is that twice the writer calls the Spirit of truth "He." What that means is that the Spirit of truth is God the Holy Spirit. Therefore, if one becomes an enemy of truth, whether consciously or subconsciously, that person is an enemy of God.

Deception is rooted in lies, which is why Jesus calls Satan the *"father of lies"* (John 8:44 [NLT]). He can deceive you and keep you in bondage to an ungodly or unhealthy soul tie. If the enemy can't destroy you by way of deception, he will try to get you to fall by way of ignorance.

It's easy for Satan to deceive the body of Christ and nonbelievers when they haven't made it a priority to grow in the knowledge of God as their lifestyle. The word "ignorance" means "a lack of knowledge, or a lack of information." Satan preys on a person's freedom when they lack the information needed to gain or keep that freedom. For every believer who is a part of the body of Christ, growing in God must be a daily goal. When the body of Christ comes into the revelation of this one conviction—that freedom is not a one-time event; freedom is a lifestyle—it will destroy the kingdom of darkness.

The apostle Peter admonishes believers in the body of Christ to grow in the knowledge of God (2 Peter 3:18). You can't grow in the knowledge of God if you're not willing to develop and grow in understanding the Word of God. The more you learn and understand about the Word of God, the easier it will be for you to identify the deception of the enemy and then not fall for his lies. All of hell loves to see a believer in Christ with an apathetic attitude toward growing in the understanding of the Word of God because apathy will keep a person in ignorance. That's why the Bible says, *"My people are destroyed for lack of knowledge"* (Hosea 4:6). What you don't know about ungodly and unhealthy soul ties is exactly what the enemy will use against you to keep you in bondage and eventually destroy you.

If the enemy can't deceive you or capitalize on your ignorance, then another tool he will use is temptation. The word "temptation" is defined as "the desire to do something—especially something wrong or unwise." In Kurt's story, he was the victim of a wrong and unwise desire. The deception behind his decision to leave his college sweetheart did not come to light until 18 years later. Kurt did not value self-control; therefore, he came to me broken, confused, and empty. The enemy will not tempt you with what you're not attracted to; rather, he will always tempt you with what you are accustomed to.

Kurt's deception and ignorance, both weaknesses in which he was easily tempted, led him into a state of unfulfillment. Anytime unhealthy desires are not controlled, expect discouragement, defeat, and depression. Another way to define temptation is the pressure applied to ungodly thinking and lustful feelings. Kurt couldn't resist the pressure of getting into a sexual relationship with his coworker. Therefore, to this day, Kurt is wrestling with regret for leaving his college sweetheart for a coworker who left him for another man.

Don't forget that the enemy comes to steal, kill and destroy (John 10:10). One of the most common ways he does this is through ungodly and unhealthy relationships. I'm thoroughly convinced and fully persuaded that Satan doesn't know your future¾that would mean that he's omniscient (all-knowing), which he is not; only Jesus Christ is all-knowing¾but I do believe that he carefully studies our patterns.

Satan doesn't have to know your future when he knows your patterns. Anytime there is not a consistent flow of growth in your life, all the enemy must do is identify what you like, and how you like it. For most people—especially single, broken, disappointed, and desperate people, as well as those who feel unloved and unaccepted—all he must do is to put someone in front of them who may act as if they would love to get to know them intimately. Even if these people realize that the person who wants into their lives is not good for them, they will succumb, due to the lack of love in their lives.

In *the Secret of the Soul Tie*, you will discover a biblical foundation for soul ties, and you'll read firsthand experiences with soul ties. You'll learn what a soul tie is, and how to tell if you're tied. You'll understand the difference between an ungodly soul tie and an unhealthy soul tie. You'll unearth the secrets that keep you tied. You'll learn the tools to untie yourself. Even after you finish reading this book, you'll keep it close as a reference to stay free.

A lot of books and sermons on soul ties give information and truth. What we know is that truth leads to freedom, but what you might not understand is that there are different dimensions of freedom. Jesus said, *"You shall know the truth, and the truth shall make you free ... therefore, if the Son sets you free, you shall be free indeed"* (John 8:31–34 [NKJV]). This tells me that there's a difference between being free and being "free indeed." You may wonder what determines the difference between a person being free and being free indeed; it is the next level of truth. You may have a level of freedom, but if you want the next level of freedom, then this book will give you the next level of truth.

I hope you're ready for the ride. If so, then let's learn about the secrets of the soul tie.

PART ONE
THE BIRTHING

CHAPTER 1
MY STORY

FOR 27 YEARS, I went by my street name, Butch. The story my family tells me, is that one day, when I was a few months old, my aunt took me to the doctor, and he looked at me, and called me, "Butch". No one ever asked him why. The name was never given a meaning. It just stuck to me, and until the age of 27, Butch is what people called me. In retrospect, I like to think it was because God always knew, He would change my name.

Today, I go by James D. Edwards. It's a privilege to be the Senior Pastor at Transforming Faith Christian Center in Houston, Texas. I'm originally from Florence, Alabama. My father was killed in 1983, when I was four years old. My mom struggled with addictions until I was 17. My grandmother on my mom's side raised me.

When I was 10 years old, my grandmother developed heart failure. Therefore, I was forced to live with my mother. It felt like every single day, I faced verbal, mental, and physical abuse. On many occasions when she was under the influence of drugs, my mother told me that I was the worst mistake she ever made.

While living with my mom, the dysfunction increased. Mom's addiction to drugs and alcohol brought the street life into our home. I saw, heard, and experienced things as a child that normal 10-year-old kids shouldn't be and aren't normally exposed to. Today, my mother and I have reconciled, but it doesn't omit the things that I endured.

At the age of 12, I had a promising future on the football field, but because I was a troubled child, the misfortune of my unruly behavior followed me every day into the classroom. It got so bad that my mom took me off the football team. My childhood dreams were shattered.

My grandmother died in December 1991, and I felt like my life was over. My granny was gone, and I couldn't play football. Nothing important was left, so I declared, "If I can't make it to the NFL or the NBA, then I'll just sell dope for the rest of my life."

At the age of 15, I sold my first piece of crack cocaine. By the time I was 18, I was transporting drugs from Florence, Alabama, to Detroit, Michigan. At the age of 20, I bought my first kilo of cocaine—36 ounces which is a drug dealer's dream —for $26K. As a result, most people in my neighborhood treated me like a celebrity. For the first time in my life, I felt accepted, appreciated, and affirmed because I was getting all that I had ever wanted from my family and friends—love.

Four years later, I boarded a flight to Houston, Texas, with $84K cash in my possession. The plan was to buy five kilos of cocaine and bring it back on the Greyhound bus. Surprisingly, the guy I was buying the drugs from, whipped out a gun, aimed it at my face, and pulled the trigger. The gun did not fire. Though he robbed me of the $84K, by the grace of God, I got away with my life.

After experiencing such a traumatic event, most people would've changed their lives, but not me. I took things to the next level. Simply because I felt invincible after that situation.

Two years later, on August 1, 2005, the FBI and the DEA had enough of me. The federal government arrested me and indicted me on the charges of conspiracy to attempt to deliver, and conspiracy to attempt to possess 50-150 kilos of cocaine and 2,000 pounds of marijuana. After they wrapped me in a federal conspiracy with 26 other affiliates, not only were they trying to convict me on drug charges, but also to involve me in two different homicides. The victims were my family members. I didn't have anything to do with either of the murders, and eventually my name was cleared.

By the mercy of God, I stood before Judge Sharon Blackburn inside the Hugo Black Federal Courthouse in Birmingham, Alabama, on April 17, 2006. That was the day that she sentenced me to eight years in federal prison.

My life, as I knew it, was over. In prison I had none of the "normal" distractions, interruptions, or interferences of my lifestyle. No longer could I run from the truth. No longer could I run from my past. Most importantly, no longer could I run from myself. I had no choice but to entertain the thoughts that were always running through my mind, but I never stopped to ponder them. I was forced to face the reality that if I returned to society with my same destructive mentality, the next time I got caught I would receive a prison sentence of life without parole.

Therefore, I started entertaining the questions of growth. Four questions continuously rolled around in my head: Who am I? Why am I here? What should I be doing with my life? Where am I going? Truly, I wanted to change my life, but unfortunately, I didn't know how.

When I arrived at the Atlanta Federal Prison Camp, I saw many illegal activities: cell phones, laptops, free-world clothing, and inmates paying correctional officers to allow prisoners to leave the prison for a few hours. It didn't take long before I was indulging in prison-yard crimes.

Around that time, my girlfriend Jessica was still living in my apartment in Atlanta. I forced her to sneak contraband into the prison when she visited me. Jessica would also pick me up, so I could leave and spend a few hours with her late at night. I had been at the federal prison camp in Atlanta for only three months when I snuck out on a Saturday night in October. Believe it or not, but the prison authorities caught me. By the grace of God, I made it back to the prison grounds without being apprehended by a police officer. If I had gotten caught off the prison grounds, I could have been sentenced to an extra five years in federal prison.

As soon as the officers discovered I was back in my cubicle, they put me in handcuffs and locked me in the Special Housing Unit. The Special Housing Unit is a prison inside of prison. I will never forget the night when they locked me in that one-man cell. It was 2:34 AM. As soon as I stepped into the cell, I dropped onto the bed. Instantly, I heard a still, small voice say, *"You're exactly where you need to be."*

It felt like the walls were closing in on me. A panic attack hit. My heart pounded in my chest. I was sweating and chilled at the same time. I fought to breathe.

Immediately, I cried out to God with the sincerest prayer I'd ever prayed in my life. As I lay face down on the floor, I said, "Lord, I'm tired! If You will just show me what I'm created for, if You will just show me why I'm here, then I'll give up everything! I'll give up the dope game; I'll give up the fast money; I'll give up the fame, and I'll give up all the women! If You just show me what I'm created for, God, then I'll give it all up!"

I continued to pray that prayer for the next few days. Then one day, I received a book in the mail from one of my aunts—*Your Best Life Now* by Joel Osteen. The first chapter's title is "Enlarge Your Vision." Osteen's message is that until you can see yourself being someone different and doing something different internally, you'll never get the opportunity to experience it externally. If you cannot see yourself owning a business internally, then you'll never own a business externally. If you can't see yourself living in a house on a hill internally, then you'll never experience living in a house on a hill externally.[1]

For the first time in my life, I understood the principle of vision. That's when I closed the book and said aloud, "Lord, I've never seen myself doing anything but selling dope. Lord, please show me what I was created for."

I sat, deep in thought. A minute later, I heard a still small voice whisper to me, *"Keep reading this chapter."*

So, I opened the book and read Chapter 1 again. Then again. After reading Chapter 1 about three times in a row, I tried to move onto Chapter 2, "Raising Your Level of Expectancy," but something kept pulling me back to Chapter 1. Suddenly, in the middle of about the eighth read, something happened. It felt like my spirit and soul left my body and went to this huge colosseum.

In the colosseum, I was standing at a podium in front of a large crowd. As I look down to my right, I saw my grandmother (Dad's mom), my mom, my aunt, and my daughter looking at me. Then I turned to my left and saw my two uncles wearing white suits. Last, I looked down at myself. I was wearing a pure white two-piece linen suit. In an instant, I was transported back into my cell, reading the book.

Was I losing my mind? The first thought that came to me was, *God is trying to tell me something.* Immediately, the next thought was, *Fool, you are losing your mind in this one-man cell!* I jumped up from the bed, ran to the door, and pounded on it.

An inmate orderly was outside my door, mopping the floor, when he heard me beating on my cell door for help. He dropped his mop and ran to my door, screaming, "Bro! You alright? What's wrong, man?"

"Man, please get the correctional officer! I think I'm about to lose my mind!" I yelled.

The orderly dashed up the hall to get the correctional officer. A minute later, they came back. The correctional officer opened the door. The smile on his face was incongruous with not only the surroundings but also my terror. "You good, man? What's going on?" he said.

I was trying to get the words out when he laughed. That's when I knew I wasn't about to tell him what I had just experienced.

"Hey, man! Ain't you that dude who was escaping down at the prison camp? Yeah, that's you," the officer said. "Stop crying, partner. This is what happens to people who try to play the system; the hole ends up playing them. Man up, bro. You'll be alright."

He slammed the door in my face. I heard the lock engage, and his footsteps as he walked away. I didn't know what to think. So, I prayed, asking God to protect my mind.

That night, they cut off all the lights at nine, and I was horrified. Whenever they turn the lights off in the special housing unit, it gets so dark that you can't even see your hand in front of your face.

I dozed off. I hadn't been asleep for five minutes when the scene I had earlier became my dream. I held a microphone to my mouth. The funny thing about the dream was that I knew I was preaching, but I couldn't hear myself saying anything. The crowd was roaring, and I felt my auntie hitting me on my back, saying, "Boy, you better preach!"

Instantly I was awake. I sat on the edge of the bed and spoke with a trembling voice, "God, are you calling me to preach?"

Seconds later, I heard a voice inside me say, *"What is the thing about you that everybody hates?"* I tried to figure it out, but I couldn't put my finger on it. About five seconds, later the voice responded, *"It's your mouth."*

Instantly, I recalled three events from my past. First, my mom was taking me to school one morning after I had been suspended for three days. She was giving me a pep talk before I walked into school. "What's wrong with you? Why can't you act like all the other kids? Why do you always have to be disobedient and get in trouble?"

"Ma! The only reason I got into a fight was because all the kids be saying that you and your friends be stealing all my clothes, and they say y'all are crackheads."

My mom slapped me across my mouth. "Shut up, bastard. I can't stand your mouth!"

The next instance took place when I was 20 years old. I was with my aunt when she was buying my first Cadillac Escalade.

While she was in the finance office, signing the paperwork for the truck, I ran inside the office, waving $15K cash in my hand, saying, "Auntie! Put this down on the truck, so my payments won't be so high."

She looked at me and shouted, "Boy, get out of here. I can't stand your mouth!"

The last instance happened a couple of months before the feds arrested me. I was sitting at the table with an ex-girlfriend who was having dinner with her coworkers. At the perfect time, I took over the conversation. I started boasting and bragging about all the things I had been doing and buying. I told them about all the money I had, all the cars I had, and how I was a neighborhood celebrity. That's when my ex-girlfriend stopped me and said, "Shut up, boy! I can't stand your mouth! You talk like a girl, and you talk too much!"

Then that still small voice spoke. *It ain't nothing wrong with talking too much; you're just talking about the wrong thing.*

In an instant, I knew that something had shifted in my life. Right at that moment, God gave me my purpose.

I decided to give God all my life.

The next morning, I woke up and started reading the Bible. It seemed like everything I was reading stuck to me like glue. As I read the stories, it was like I was inside of a movie, experiencing everything I was reading. I felt the passion for the Word of God accelerating inside of me. My hunger for knowing deepened, and my commitment to being 100 percent obedient to the Word of God was being solidified every day.

As time progressed, the Word kept changing me at a rapid pace. Satan saw it. He decided to expose my weaknesses.

I CREATED A SOUL TIE

I'll never forget Memorial Day weekend, 2007. I hadn't seen my girlfriend Jessica since December of the previous year, right before the Bureau of Prisons shipped me from Atlanta to Big Spring, Texas, for my disciplinary transfer. On the weekend Jessica came to Big Spring to visit me, I had a four-day weekend of interaction because it was Memorial Day.

As soon as she stepped into the visitation room, I gave her a big kiss and a long hug. We sat down, and I looked into her eyes with the strongest intensity of love I had ever felt for her. Mentally, I was in another dimension because I hadn't seen her in a while. My emotions were stronger and deeper.

I was excited, happy, and grateful to be in Jessica's presence. I immediately told her about every detail of growth I had experienced since the last time we had seen each other. I shared with her about preaching my first sermon. Then I cast vision after vision about how great our lives were going to be when I was released from prison. I broke down every book I had read. Because she was quiet the entire time, I believed that my words were penetrating and making an impact inside her heart. The visit was supposed to be a dialogue between us, but I turned it into a monologue.

My total conversation consisted of Jesus, Jesus, and more about Jesus! I was on fire. The only time I allowed her to talk was when I asked her if she was being faithful to me. But she never addressed that question. We discussed a few things about her life, but not too much. My focus was to convince Jessica that I was a changed man, and I aimed to make sure I said everything I thought would sway her to stay by my side while I remained in prison for the next five years.

During those four days, I shoved Jesus down her throat and tried to force her to find a church. I tried to strengthen our connection by any means necessary, but I didn't know Jessica's true motive for coming to see me until the last day of our four-day visit. Sadly, on that Memorial Day Monday, I entered the visitation room, excited to be with Jessica—until I saw a disturbed look on her face. I hugged her, ignored her dark countenance, and tried to pick up from where we had left off the day before.

About a minute into my lecture, Jessica stopped me with a statement that shook me to the core of my being. "Butch, when are you going to shut up talking about you and listen, so you can hear about me? I don't care that you keep trying to prove to me that you have changed. Ever since I walked into this visitation room, you have been talking about yourself, and what you've got going on in your life. Yeah, I think you've changed a little bit, but who don't change when they go to prison? Everybody gets out of prison with all these big dreams, talking about what they are going to do, and how they're going to do it. All that stuff that you are saying right now don't even matter to me until you get out, live on the street a couple of years, and prove it because if you were all that changed, then you would still be in Atlanta, and I wouldn't have to be catching rides all the way here to Texas with people I don't even know! So, save your breath and listen to what I have going on."

It wasn't so much about what she said that hurt me, but it was how she said it that sent a knife into my heart. It felt like a deep gut check of rejection, and I didn't know how to handle it. I knew it was rejection because I was so familiar with that from my past. I didn't want to accept it.

"Butch listen. Ain't nothing going right for me. I got fired from my job, the people at the apartment complex have sent me an eviction notice, and they're saying if I don't pay the rent by Thursday, they are going to put me out. On top of all that, I wrecked your Escalade a couple of weeks ago, and I don't have any money to pay the deductible for the insurance company to get it fixed."

"What! How did you do that?" I raised my voice in disbelief.

"I was driving home one night, and I just had a wreck. It was an accident," Jessica said sadly.

"How bad is the truck damaged? What's wrong with it?" I asked.

"It's bad. I couldn't drive it home after the wreck, and the people had to send the wrecker truck to tow it to the Cadillac dealership."

We sat in silence until she continued. "I don't have a car to get around town. I don't have a job, and I'm about to get put out of the apartment. Instead of you worrying about yourself right now, show me how you're going to help me."

Confusion assailed me. She was preparing to use me and then leave me, but I didn't want to accept it. "Where is your Lincoln LS? You don't have it anymore?"

"Nope. The people came and repossessed it a couple of months ago."

"Why didn't you tell me when it happened?" I asked.

"Because you already got enough on your plate right now, and I wasn't going to add any more stress while you're locked up. At first, I wasn't tripping because I still had the Escalade, but now, since I wrecked it, I'm messed up. I don't know what I'm about to do with my life. I can't go back to Alabama because my friends and family will be talking about me if I have to go back and live with my mother," Jessica said.

She had me in tears. Her words tore me up. I felt sorry for her while knowing that she was trying to manipulate me. I contemplated a few things I could arrange from prison to help her get back on her feet. Before I could voice any ideas, she spoke. "I know that you are going to make a way for me some kind of way. Butch, please don't let me down."

With a heavy heart and a focused mind, I looked at her in the eyes with every ounce of love I had in me. "Don't I always come through for you in the clutch? I'm going to show you just how much I love you."

A few hours later, visitation ended. Tears filled our eyes and trailed down our cheeks as we said goodbye. We locked pinky fingers and made vows to each other, promising that nothing and nobody would ever separate us or come between the bond we shared. As soon as the words left out of my mouth, that's when I felt something touch me inside.

As Jessica walked out of the visitation room, that still, small voice came to me. *This is your last time seeing Jessica as your girl-friend. She is about to leave you.*

To be honest, I ignored the voice because my heart was knitted to her. Plus, I didn't want to face the truth of Jessica leaving me while I was in one of the most vulnerable seasons of my life. A few months later, after my aunt had paid off the truck, I signed the title over to Jessica. Then she crushed my heart by not keeping her vow.

One day I called her phone and another guy answered it. My heart shattered, even though I knew it was coming. For the next couple of years, I couldn't understand how I could be physically disconnected from a relationship while Jessica was actively still living inside of me. Eventually God would show me that I had created an ungodly soul tie. He didn't leave me hanging because he also showed me how to sever and outgrow the ungodly soul tie.

Get your pen and paper ready. Follow me closely if you're ready to be introduced to the next level of growth.

CHAPTER 2

WHO AM I?

THE TRICHOTOMY of mankind (composed of spirit, soul, and body) is one of the most misunderstood, misapplied, misused, and undervalued teachings in Western church culture today. One reason is that most people have been led to believe that their spirits and souls are the same. If you study the Bible intending to determine this truth, you will discover that your spirit and soul are separate. This is extremely important when it comes to breaking a soul tie because what you don't know can become the tool (ignorance) the enemy uses to keep you in bondage to the soul tie.

Therefore, if you are going to break free, you must make it a priority to become best friends with biblical interpersonal knowledge. I heard the late great Dr. Myles Monroe say, "The greatest revelation of life, is not discovering the truth about something else or someone else, but the greatest revelation of life is when you discover the truth about yourself." When you come into a great understanding of how and why God created and designed each person on the face of this planet, that's when you understand how a person can be tied not only to someone else but also to something else.

The Bible says, *"And the Lord God formed man of the dust of the ground and breathed into his nostrils the breath of life, and man became a living soul"* (Genesis 2:7). The Hebrew word for the phrase "the breath of life" is *ruach* and refers to the spirit of life.[1] When God created the first man, Adam, He created his spirit to be intertwined with His Own Spirit. Then man became a living soul. At that point, the spirit of man and the soul of man were housed in the body of man.

One of the most powerful and enlightening revelations I've come to understand is the reality of the trichotomy of mankind. The trichotomy of mankind reveals that all people are spirit beings. We have a soul that exists within a body. The Bible says that *"God is a Spirit"* (John 4:24). According to Genesis 2:7, *"God breathed the spirit of life into man,"* and according to Genesis 1:26, *"Humans were made in the image of God."* Therefore, all humans are spirit beings; God is a Spirit, and humans come from God.

Because we are called human beings, it's easy to think we are earthly beings having a spiritual experience. According to the Bible, we are spiritual beings having an earthly experience.

The first man, Adam, was created as a perfect spirit, with a perfect soul and a perfect body. He experienced the totality of godly love, power, freedom, and truth. Adam and Eve lived in a perfect world, in which nothing was missing, nothing was broken, and nothing was lost. They walked with the Voice of the Lord in the cool of the day, every day. They experienced unhindered fellowship with their Heavenly Father for a season. They experienced what it felt like to have complete dominion over the fish in the sea, the fowl in the air, and all the creeping things upon the Earth.

Adam was given only one instruction: *"And the Lord God commanded the man, saying, 'Of every tree of the garden, thou mayest freely eat, but of the Tree of the Knowledge of Good and Evil, thou shalt not eat of it, for on the day that thou eatest thereof, thou shalt surely die"* (Genesis 2:16–17).

God the Father gave Adam an opportunity to exercise his free will and prove his honor to the Voice of God. God the Father made Adam fully aware of the consequences that came with disobedience. It was one word: *death.* The word "death" in Hebrew is *mut* and conveys the idea of separation. As soon as Adam rebelled against the instructions of God the Father, the Spirit of God that was inside Adam released Himself from Adam. That's when the nature of Satan found his home inside the spirit of Adam. In other words, there was an exchange that happened: God's Spirit exited man, and Satan's spirit entered him.

At that point, what Adam knew as the perfect place on Earth became his personal hell because Adam had separated himself from the Spirit of God. Consequently, anytime that anyone or anything is separated from the Spirit of God, they exist in a state of hell.

God the Father created the Earth for Adam and his descendants to have total dominion and authority over. After that one act of disobedience, Adam gave his dominion and authority to the hand of Satan, but Adam's treason and rebellion did not catch God the Father by surprise. Don't forget that God the Father is omniscient, meaning he's all-knowing. God the Father is omnipresent, meaning he is always everywhere. God the Father is also omnipotent, meaning he is all-powerful. Therefore, He already had a Plan B in place.

God the Father announced, *"And the Lord God said unto the serpent, 'Because thou hast done this, thou art cursed above all cattle, and above every beast of the field; upon thy belly shalt thou go, and dust thou shalt eat all the days of thy life, and I will put enmity between thee and the woman, and between thy seed and her seed; it shall bruise thy head, and thou shalt bruise his heel"* (Genesis 3:14–15).

This was the Plan B that God the Father put into action. God knew that man had willingly released his spirit into the hands of Satan, and if God the Father were going to retrieve humankind, then He would have to redeem the spirit of humans by way of a perfect and sinless man, whose blood would have to be without spot or blemish.

The word "redeem" means "to buy back." The only way to buy back humankind was by way of the payment of sinless blood. That's why forty-two generations later, God the Father wrapped God the Son (Jesus) in human flesh and placed him in the seed of a virgin woman, Mary. God the Son was all divinity traveling down the birth canal of humanity. When he was brought forth, being 100% God and 100% man, the world knew something was special about him, but they couldn't fully identify what it was.

For 33 years, Jesus walked the Earth without sin. He came to the Earth to destroy the works of the devil (1 John 3:8) and to pay the penalty for the sins of all humankind. Why would he do such a thing? Because Adam hadn't fulfilled his obedience to God, so Jesus had to fulfill it in his place.

When Adam ate from the Tree of the Knowledge of Good and Evil, his nature became one with the nature of Satan, and so did all his offspring. Therefore, the entire human race is born in sin because every person comes from the seed of Adam (in the natural). As the Bible says, *"Yielding seed after his kind"* (Genesis 1:12). That means Adam's own kind is sin because when he rebelled against the instructions of God, the Holy Spirit exited Adam and the nature of Satan (i.e., sin) entered him.

Even though Jesus was born of a woman, the Bible said that Jesus was conceived of the Holy Ghost. In other words, the Holy Spirit supplied the seed, becoming the Father of Jesus (Matthew 1:20). Therefore, the blood of Jesus, whom Mary carried, was the same blood that would be the atonement for her sins as well as the sins of the entire world.

After Jesus fulfilled his earthly mission, he willingly laid down his life to die. His death was a sin-offering that was the substitutionary atonement to give humankind the opportunity for the Spirit of God to come back and live inside the spirit of each person. This is why Paul wrote, *"But what does it say? 'The word is near you, in your mouth and in your heart'* [i.e., the word of faith which we preach] *that if you confess with your mouth the Lord Jesus and believe in your heart that God has raised Him from the dead, you will be saved. For with the heart, one believes unto righteousness, and with the mouth, confession is made unto salvation"* (Romans 10:8–10 [NKJV]).

To receive salvation, the preliminary requirements are to hear the gospel, receive it, confess that Jesus is Lord, and believe it in your heart. Then God the Holy Spirit comes into your heart and regenerates your spirit. At that point, you become a son or a daughter of God. Anytime you see the words "spirit," "heart," or "inner man" in the scriptures, it's referring to the spirit of the person.

When you confess and receive Christ into your spirit and your heart, God the Holy Spirit comes inside you, and He becomes one with your spirit (1 Corinthians 6:17). At that moment, salvation happens in your spirit, not in your soul. This is important to know because many believers don't know how they are saved, and they don't know where God lives in them. According to Ephesians 2:8, through faith in Jesus' death, burial, and resurrection, Heaven releases grace, and God the Holy Spirit comes to live within your spirit: *"That if any man be in Christ, He is a new creature"* (2 Corinthians 5:17).

This is extremely powerful because God the Holy Spirit is the only One who can save any person on the face of this planet. You're not saved by your charitable deeds; you're not saved by your monetary gifts; you're not saved because you feed the homeless; you're not saved because your parents are pastors of a church. You are saved because of God's grace that comes upon you by your faith in Christ Jesus.

Salvation is your way to spend eternity in heaven, but heaven comes to live inside of your born-again spirit. When the Pharisees asked Jesus when the kingdom of God would come, He answered, *"The Kingdom of God does not come with observation, nor will they say, 'See here!' or 'See there!' For indeed, the Kingdom of God is within you"* (Luke 17:20-21 [NKJV]).

According to Jesus, the kingdom of God is within you. You might wonder how that is possible. Romans 14:17 tells us: *"For the Kingdom of God is not in eating and drinking, but righteousness and peace and joy in the Holy Spirit"* (NKJV).

After I read that, a bomb went off inside me. The Bible says plainly that the Kingdom of God is in the Holy Spirit, and the Holy Spirit lives inside every child of God. Therefore, it's correct to say, "I know I am saved because the God of the Universe lives inside me!" You can also say, "I know I'm saved because the Kingdom of God is inside me."

When God is in your spirit, the kingdom of God is in your spirit and your spirit is born again. That's why your spirit, your heart, and your inward man are brand-new in Christ Jesus.

Here is the amazing part: Salvation has benefits on the Earth. The word "salvation" comes from the Greek word *soteria*, and the Hebrew word *Yehoshua*. These words mean "wholeness, healing, welfare, prosperity, victory, and deliverance." Therefore, salvation encompasses every area of life: personal, financial, career, marriage, family, education, home, and spiritual.

Let's study some of the salvation words.

WHOLENESS

Wholeness means that nothing is missing; nothing is broken, and nothing is lost in your spirit. When the Kingdom of God comes into your spirit, nothing is missing, broken, or lost. John 4:4 confirms this: *"Greater is He that is in you, than he that is in the world."*

When the woman with the plague of blood touched the hem of Jesus' garment, immediately the flow of blood was dried up. She felt it in her body that she was healed of that plague:

> "And Jesus, immediately knowing within
> Himself that virtue had gone out of Him,
> turned Him about in the press and said, 'Who
> touched my clothes?' And His disciples said
> unto Him, 'Thou seest the multitude
> thronging Thee, and sayest Thou, "Who
> touched me?"' And He looked around to see
> she who had done this thing, but the woman,
> fearing and trembling, knowing what was

done in her, came and fell down before him
and told him all the truth, and He said unto
her, 'Daughter, thy faith has made thee
whole. Go in peace and be whole of thy
plague.'"

— MARK 5: 30-34

HEALING

Jesus made this woman whole not only in her body but also in her spirit. When He made her spirit whole, her self-value, self-acceptance, self-belief, and self-confidence were restored. When Jesus healed her body, he took away the plague, infirmity, disease, or sickness that was afflicting her earthly lifestyle.

The word "healed" comes from the Greek word *iaomai*, which means "to heal, to cure, and to restore to bodily health." One of the first demonstrations of the Gospel of Jesus Christ is healing: *"How God anointed Jesus of Nazareth with the Holy Ghost and with power, who went about doing good and healing all who were oppressed of the devil; for God was with him"* (Acts 10:38).

As soon as Jesus Christ began His ministry, He chose four disciples to follow him. The first thing He did was to go throughout all of Galilee, teaching in the synagogues, preaching the gospel of the kingdom, and healing all kinds of sickness and all kinds of diseases among the people (Matt. 4:23). Everyone who came to him for healing received it.

One reason the gospel is demonstrated through healing is to show that the Kingdom of God is the most superior Kingdom on this Earth. If the same Spirit that raised Jesus from the grave lives within you, then that same Spirit will heal you and others through you because you are a joint heir in Jesus Christ (Romans 8:10–17).

WELFARE

Biblically, *welfare* refers to heavenly protection and the peace of God. Did you know that God assigned heavenly angels to protect and help usher you into your divine destiny? The author of Hebrews wrote, *"But to which of the angels said he at any time, 'Sit at my right hand until I make your enemies your footstool?' Are they not all ministering spirits, sent forth to minister for them who shall be heirs of salvation?"* (Hebrews 1:13–14).

You have thousands of angels waiting on you to activate them to go into the realm of the spirit, apprehend what is yours, and position you to receive it in the natural. Not only is your welfare about heavenly protection, but it's also about heavenly peace. Jesus is called "the Prince of Peace," who can fill your heart with joy and peace. That's why the Bible says, *"Therefore, being justified by faith, we have peace with God through our Lord Jesus Christ"* (Romans 5:1). Peace is not just the absence of chaos; peace is the presence of God the Holy Spirit. He is the Spirit of Peace.

PROSPERITY

The word "prosperity" is one many people hate to hear about but would love to have. The apostle John prayed for Gaius, *"Beloved, I wish above all things that thou mayest prosper and be in health, even as thy soul prospereth"* (3 John 2). He was praying that Gaius and all believers would be blessed to have more than enough resources, so they could fulfill the plan and purpose of God and their lives.

Prosperity simply means more than enough. God wants you to have not only more than enough money but also more than enough joy, peace, relationships, ideas, and resources to fulfill your God-given assignment. As you are doing that, he wants you to have more than enough wisdom, peace, love, strength, favor, vision, and faith so that nothing is missing, nothing is broken, and nothing is lost.

God's idea of blessing His children, or other people, financially flows through the children of God who are blessed financially. How can you give a family member or friend or a brother in Christ any amount of money when you don't have it? Anytime you're in lack, debt, or scarcity, the enemy can tempt you to do things outside of your godly identity to meet your needs.

Therefore, the tools of the enemy are poverty, lack, and scarcity. If he can cement you in this place, you will compromise your commitment to God. On the other hand, the will of God and the heart of salvation for every child of God are for us to have more than enough to bless the people who are struggling. It takes finances to live, so why would God not want you to live in financial freedom?

God doesn't have a problem with his children having more than enough. He just doesn't want them to develop "pride" in having more than enough. When the pride of more than enough has you, you will act in arrogance and self-righteousness. At that point, what was intended to be a blessing to you will become a burden.

VICTORY

The fifth aspect of salvation is victory. God deposited victory into the DNA of salvation because he knew that this life is a war. As you're reading this book, the chances are high that you're in a war with emotions that are trying to make you give into feelings of negativity. Allow me to remind you what Jesus said in John 16:33: *"In the world, you will have tribulations; but be of good cheer because I have overcome the world"* (NKJV). The revelation behind this scripture tells us that in this life, we have to fight. This is why Paul wrote to Timothy, *"Fight the good fight of faith; lay hold on eternal life"* (1 Timothy 6:12 NKJV). Yes, we have to fight, but through Jesus Christ, we've already come out victorious.

One fruit that comes from the fight with negative emotions is self-control. After you win one fight, you learn that you can win future fights. You don't have to react to the attacks of the enemy as one who hasn't had a victory but as one who already has victory!

Anytime you've won a battle, you're equipped to approach a new battle with boldness, confidence, faith, and full assurance because you have a history of defeating the enemy. That means when the problem comes, you're not terrified, you're not thinking negative thoughts, and you're not seeing it through the eyes of a loser.

"We are more than conquerors" (Romans 8:37) informs us that we are fully equipped with everything we need to defeat the enemy. Plus, we can learn the fresh wisdom that comes from battle. In this book, you're learning not only how to defeat the enemy but also how to help other people going through similar situations to defeat the enemy.

DELIVERANCE

The sixth and final aspect of salvation is deliverance. Jesus came to Earth to set us free from the penalty of sin. Freedom has always been God's absolute priority for all humankind. Before the creation of man in Genesis 1:26, God spoke the purpose of our free will into our DNA. He said, *"Let Us make man in Our image, after Our likeness, and let them have dominion."* I want to focus on the phrase "let them." These two words imply that God released His authority into the hands of the people of His creation so that they could choose how to rule or govern, absent from the sovereignty of God. The phrase "let them" exchanges God's sovereignty for humanity's responsibility to choose freely.

Adam named the animals, choosing the names himself, rather than God telling him what to name them. Adam had total control over all the Earth when he was in his perfect, sinless state, but as soon as Adam willfully sinned, he gave his rights of rulership and dominion to Satan and his demonic thugs. At that point, Satan reversed and perverted everything that God had originally purposed for humankind on the Earth.

In the beginning, God told Adam to rule over the Earth, but He never told him to rule over people. However, as soon as Satan took charge, he caused the Earth to rule over humans, and he turned the people against one another. One example of how he did this can be found in coca leaves. Cocaine is made from coca leaves. Cocaine is highly addictive and creates havoc in the lives of addicts and their families. Cocaine is a perversion of the leaves' healing elements, as they are used to relieve altitude sickness by chewing them or making tea with them—not to get high. Any time coca leaves are abused or misused, cocaine controls people, instead of people controlling the coca leaves or cocaine.

God's heart was always for a people to love others, not for one person to use strength as a way of overpowering a weaker person. When that happens, bondage is the result. Bondage was never the plan of God. *Ungodly soul ties are bondage.*

God sent Jesus to deliver us from the hands of Satan and out of the bondage of ungodly soul ties. God coded deliverance into salvation so that all His children would always have a way of escape from anything that had control over them.

Salvation takes place in your spirit, but to experience the fullness of salvation, what's in your spirit must flow into your mind. It's one thing to be free in your spirit, but it's something different to be free in your soul.

I exposed you to earthly salvation, so you would know what God's heart is for every born-again believer who lives on Earth. The trick of the enemy is to connect you to an unhealthy or ungodly soul tie so that it produces brokenness in your life. Becoming one with a person who betrays you, neglects you, or rejects you leads to brokenness. Living in brokenness will cement you in fear and insecurity. Plus, it will rob you of your peace. The ungodly soul tie will come into your life and defeat you. If that person gets enough power over you, then they can send you into financial debt. All this bondage that comes from an ungodly soul tie is designed to steal, kill, and destroy your access to earthly salvation.

Don't think for one second that you can't experience such heartbreak, or that it won't leave you sick. If you don't sever the soul tie, you'll be on your way to Heaven but living in hell right here on Earth.

CHAPTER 3
THE SOUL MAN

IN THE PREVIOUS CHAPTER, we learned that human beings are made up of three parts: spirit, soul, and body. We did a thorough investigation of the spirit of the person that was created in the image of God before the first man, Adam, chose to sin. Remember, when we say the spirit, we're also talking about the heart and the inner man. In Scripture, the heart, the inner man, and the spirit are interchangeable terms.

When God communicates with you and me, He does so by way of our spirits. Jesus said, "God is a Spirit" (John 4:24). God made human beings in his image, which is Spirit. Therefore, sometimes when God contacts and communicates with us, He does it from Spirit to spirit.

In our spirits, we are God-conscious, but in our souls, we are self-conscious. The first time we see the word "soul" in the Bible is in Genesis 2:7: *"And the Lord God formed man from the dust of the ground, then He breathed into his nostrils the breath of life, and man became a living soul."* The word "soul" is derived from the Hebrew word *nephesh*, which describes the faculties of the soul that causes a man to function properly on Earth. The soul is comprised of the mind, will, emotions, memory, imagination, and personality.

Let's look at each of these areas:

- **Mind:** Your brain is not your mind; your mind is your thinker. When God created the mind, it was perfect, without any defects, before sin entered the spirit, soul, or body. The mind did and still does operate when it receives words, scents, tastes, thoughts, sensations, pictures, and sounds. Whether positive or negative input, the mind tends to flow in the direction of what you hear, see, sense, taste, feel, or say.

- **Will:** The will was and is our chooser. At creation, Adam's will (his chooser) was pure perfection in the eyes of God. Even after Adam sinned, he was free to choose whatever he wanted, without being forced to be for or against God. That is why God said, *"Let them have dominion"* (Genesis 1:26). "Let them" coming from the mouth of God is one of the strongest phrases in the Bible. As we continue to journey through this book, you'll understand just how powerful your personal choice—your free will—is to your wholeness and healing.

- **Emotions:** Emotions are your feelers. Emotions are feelings provoked by pain or pleasure. Emotions are like fire. Fire can heat a home or burn it down. When God created Adam with emotions, He didn't do it so that He could control Adam but to guide him in the direction of truth. People have both good and bad emotions, but it was never in the plan and purpose of God for a person to be led or driven by emotions.

- **Memory:** Memory is a replay of the past. It is comprised of mental pictures of what you have seen, felt, heard, smelled, and tasted. Memory is designed to draw you back to something you experienced—whether good or bad. You're not locked into using your memory to always think about something negative; you can also use your memory to remember God's goodness, and great times that produced life, joy, confidence, love, and happiness.

- **Imagination:** The imagination is the vision of a potential future reality. You can use this part of the soul to create a picture of what you want to have or happen in the future, no matter if it's positive or negative. The enemy desires for you to imagine the worst of things so that you attract the worst in your life. God created you with an imagination so you can use it to see the best of things, so you can bring the best into your life. That's why Ephesians 3:20 says, *"Never doubt God's mighty power to work in you and accomplish all this. He will achieve infinitely more than your greatest request, your most unbelievable dream, and exceed your wildest imagination!"* (TPT).

- **Personality:** Last, the personality is a combination of qualities that forms an individual's habits, ways, and character traits. Every personality is different in every person, which makes us unique and individual human beings.

The soulish realm is important to know and understand because your soul and spirit are not the same. Anytime a person gets saved, or when a person gives their life to God, the spirit becomes new, but the soul is still "old," as it was before salvation. In other words, thoughts, decisions, feelings, memories, imaginations, and personality do not change when a person is born again. On the other hand, the heart, spirit man, or inner man does change completely into the DNA of Jesus Christ.

When a person accepts Jesus as their personal Lord and Savior, immediately they become God's child. At this point, God chooses to see His child from his spirit to his soul and to his body. 1 Corinthians 6:17 explains why: *"He that is joined unto the Lord is one spirit."* God is a Spirit Being, and you are a spirit being; therefore, God starts everything from the spirit to the natural.

When God sees you from your spirit, he sees his spirit in you: *"That we might become the righteousness of God in Him"* (2 Corinthians 5:21 [NKJV]). Because God chooses to see you from your spirit, Jesus said, *"As many as received Him, to them He gave the power to become the sons of God"* (John 1:12).

This is so important to understand because one of the tools you'll need to break and sever an ungodly or unhealthy soul tie is your self-perception, which is the way you see yourself. We will discuss this thoroughly in the coming chapters.

My assignment is to inform how God sees you so that you can choose to see yourself the same way. Let me repeat; it is extremely important to see yourself exactly as God sees you. God sees you from your spirit because God is living inside your spirit, and your spirit is perfect. That does not mean that all your actions are perfect, but your spirit is perfect. Your soul is not perfect because it is old, but your spirit is perfect because it is new. It is a new creation. Therefore, God longs for you to see yourself from your spirit to your soul and to your body. So, when you commit to renewing your soul, you will have a reference point. In other words, your soul will see your perfect spirit, so it can start to pursue it.

It's possible to train and discipline your soul to such a profound degree that it looks like your spirit. If that was not possible, the Bible would not say that you have the mind of Christ (1 Corinthians 2:16). According to Romans 12:1-2, it's our responsibility to renew our minds so that we can prove what is that good, acceptable, and perfect will of God for our lives. We start with renewing our minds because our thoughts are the driving force that creates our emotions.

Often, once we start feeling whatever we are thinking, it won't be long before we choose in the direction of whatever we are feeling. Once we make the choice, whether godly or ungodly, the action taken tends to become repetitive. In other words, if you do something once and it feels good, you'll be tempted to do it again, whether it's godly or ungodly. If the action is repeated, it has the power to turn into a habit.

Anytime a habit is formed and exercised long enough, eventually it will become a character trait. Whatever character trait you create can become a lifestyle. Therefore, when you go back to the genesis of this entire process, you'll see how it all started from a thought. What if this sequence was started by a godly thought, word, or picture? Following this process, we would produce godly beliefs, emotions, convictions, decisions, actions, habits, traits, characters, and lifestyles.

On the other hand, when the soul is old and ungodly, a person can be a Christian because their spirit is new, and they can go to Heaven, but because their soul is old, they will live in hell on Earth. I want you to thoroughly understand this. Just because your spirit is new doesn't mean your old soul will automatically follow your new spirit. The spirit-person is God's responsibility to make new, but the soul is your responsibility to make new.

If you're like me, then you may wonder how humans got to this point. In the first two chapters of Genesis, God the Father revealed His plan and purpose for humanity.

God the Father said these words:

> "Let us make man in Our image, after Our like-ness, and let them have dominion over the fish of the sea and over the fowl of the air and over the cattle and over all the Earth and over every creeping thing that creepeth upon the Earth.' So, God created man in His own image; in the image of God, He created him; male and female, He created them, and God blessed them, and God said unto them, 'Be fruitful and multiply and replenish the Earth and subdue it and have dominion over the fish of the sea and over the fowl of the air and over every living thing that moveth upon the Earth."

> — GENESIS 1:26-28

In these verses, we see God's prophecy of how He would make humankind in His image and His likeness, and we see all the instructions that God gave to them. Next, He spoke a blessing over them to be fruitful and multiply, to replenish the Earth, and to subdue it. God created humankind with the ability to reproduce other human beings; therefore, God blessed them and instructed them to reproduce.

Don't miss this part of the reproduction cycle. God the Father put the seed principle in place (Genesis 1:12). That means that everything God created has a seed already placed in it, to reproduce after its own kind. An apple seed produces an apple tree not a cherry tree; an acorn produces an oak tree not an elm tree; a squash seed produces a squash plant not a strawberry plant. The seed principle is not limited to trees and plants; it also applies to animals and people.

In Genesis 2:7, we see the activation and demonstration of God the Father's declaration: *"And the Lord God formed man of the dust of the ground and breathed into his nostrils the breath of life, and man became a living soul."* Once again, this is why I say that every human is a three-part being. After Adam was created, God placed him in the garden of Eden to dress it and keep it. That's when the Lord God commanded the man, saying, *"Of every tree of the garden, thou mayest freely eat, but of the Tree of the Knowledge of Good and Evil, thou shalt not eat of it, for in the day that thou eatest thereof, thou shalt surely die."*

THREE TYPES OF DEATH

Genesis 2:17 is the first time we read the word "die" in the Bible. It is from the Hebrew *mut*, which we learned earlier means "separation." There are three types of death in Scripture: (1) physical death, (2) eternal death, and (3) spiritual death. In physical death, the spirit and soul leave the body so that the body can return to the dust of the ground.

The second type of death is eternal death. In this death, which follows physical death, the spirit and soul return to its Creator (God the Father), but if the Creator does not see his Spirit (Holy Spirit) intertwined with the human spirit. This person will then be separated from the Creator eternally. In other words, if a person doesn't accept Jesus as their personal Lord and Savior during their lifespan, then they will not die in Christ. Instead, they will be eternally separated from God the Father.

The third type of death is spiritual death. This occurs when a person has not accepted and anchored their faith in Jesus Christ as their Lord and Savior. Therefore, the Spirit of Christ isn't living inside this person's spirit. Consequently, they are spiritually dead because the Spirit of God is separated or disconnected from the person's spirit. That's why it's our job as Christians to lead our family, friends, and others to Jesus Christ, so they can eternally be a part of the family of God. Allow me to let you in on a little secret: If an ungodly soul tie gets the opportunity, they will usher you into spiritual, physical, and eternal death.

After God the Father commanded Adam and Eve not to eat from the Tree of the Knowledge of Good and Evil (Genesis 2:17), he announced that he would make for Adam a helpmeet (Genesis 2:20). God caused a deep sleep to come upon Adam. As Adam slept, God the Father took one of his ribs from his side and created woman from it. When Adam woke up, God the Father presented her to Adam. At that point, Adam said, *"This is now bone of my bones, and flesh of my flesh; she shall be called 'woman' because she was taken out of man"* (Genesis 2:23).

Even though God presented Eve to Adam, it was still Adam's responsibility to accept and choose her. In the next verse, God the Father made an important statement about soul ties: *"Therefore, shall a man leave his father and his mother and shall cleave unto his wife, and they shall be one flesh"* (Genesis 2:24).

Now, we will see the invasion of the most hated enemy of humankind. Satan enters the scene in the body of a serpent. *"Now, the serpent was more subtle than any beast of the field which the Lord God had made, and he said unto the woman, 'Yea, hath God said, "Ye shall not eat of every tree of the garden"?'"* (Genesis 3:1). As to how the snake could speak, I don't know, but what I can tell you is that God the Father created the Earth with laws for spiritual beings to abide. One law was that it is illegal for spiritual beings—of which Satan is one—to operate in or on the Earth unless they are inside an earthly body.

God the Father could not operate outside an earthly body; therefore, He created man and breathed His Spirit into Adam, so he could operate on the Earth through man. The adversary, Satan, Lucifer, or the accuser of the brethren—which are just a few names of the enemy—couldn't operate on the Earth unless from inside a body also. He couldn't inhabit a human body initially; therefore, he entered the body of a snake to carry out his goal of gaining control of the Earth.

As you can see, one of the most common tools the enemy uses in his quest to steal, kill, and destroy humankind is suggestion. The only way Satan can stop God's plan that flows through us on Earth is to get us moving in direct opposition to the Word of God. Therefore, he made a suggestion to Eve. His suggestion gave Eve another choice. The Bible records, *"And the woman said unto the serpent, 'We may eat of the fruit of the trees of the garden, but of the fruit of the tree which is in the midst of the garden, God hath said, 'Ye shall not eat of it; neither shall ye touch it, lest ye die'"* (Genesis 3:2-3).

Adam had passed on God's instructions to Eve before she spoke to the serpent. Adam was with Eve during the discourse, yet he never interrupted the ungodly conversation. This should be a wake-up call to men who are the heads of households. We should never allow our wives and children to have an ungodly conversation in our presence without interrupting and bringing in God's divine order.

Let's go back to Genesis 2:16-17 to review God the Father's instructions to Adam: *"And the Lord God commanded the man, saying, 'Of every tree of the garden, thou mayest freely eat, but of the Tree of the Knowledge of Good and Evil, thou shalt not eat of it, for on the day that thou eatest thereof, thou shalt surely die."*

The serpent came back with his deception by suggesting, *"You shall not surely die, for God doth know that the day you eat thereof, then your eyes shall be opened, and ye shall be as gods, knowing good and evil"* (Genesis 3:4-5).

Now, you can see how the demonic manipulation is disguised by way of demonic suggestion. The serpent's suggestion was to make the woman question her identity. According to Psalms 82:6, God said, *"I have said, ye are gods, and all of you are children of the Most High."* So, Adam and Eve were already in the god class because they were made in the image and likeness of God. Plus, human beings have free will to make choices, and the Bible says, *"The Heaven—even the heavens—are the LORD's, but the Earth hath He given to the children of men"* (Psalms 115:16). The scripture conveys that in the beginning, it was established that the heavens are the Lord's dwelling, but the Earth is humankind's dwelling and place of ruling.

As soon as Eve heard the serpent's suggestion, the operation of her soul started to manifest. Remember, this is when there was no sin on the Earth or within human beings. *"And when the woman saw that the tree was good for food, and that it was pleasant to the eyes, and a tree to be desired to make one wise, she took of the fruit thereof and did eat and gave also unto her husband with her, and he did eat"* (Genesis 3:6).

Here was the worst decision of all time. Through the operation of the soul (the mind, will, and emotions), Adam declared independence from his Source, which affected all of humankind from that point forward. It was never God's plan for human beings to live disconnected from himself, but by Adam's free will, he accepted the enemy's suggestion above remaining obedient to God's instruction. Please grasp this fact: When God created Adam and Eve, He created them with a perfect and complete soul. When they sinned against God the Father, they didn't lose their spirits, souls, or bodies; instead, their spirits were filled with the nature of Satan—sin. Instantly, their souls were contaminated with "the flesh," and their bodies were infected with sickness.

As soon as Adam disobeyed the instructions of God the Father, the Spirit of God departed out of the spirit of man, and the spirit of Satan filled the spirit of man. So instead of living his entire life with the nature of God, Adam, as a result, lived the rest of his life intertwined with the nature of Satan.

This is why the Bible says, *"And they heard the Voice of the Lord God walking in the garden in the cool of the day, and Adam and his wife hid themselves from the presence of the Lord God amongst the trees of the garden, and the Lord God called unto Adam and said unto him, 'Where art thou?'"* (Genesis 3:8-9). If Adam still had the nature of God the Father after he had sinned against the Word of God, why would he hide from the voice of the Lord? If Adam and God had walked and talked throughout the cool of the day beforehand without fear, why would the couple be afraid now?

Simply because the nature of God had separated from the sin nature that now inhabited Adam and Eve. When God called to Adam, "Adam where art thou?" it wasn't because he didn't know where Adam was; rather, it was because he wanted Adam to know that his spirit was no longer intertwined with God's Spirit.

Listen to Adam's response: *"I heard Thy voice in the garden, and I was afraid because I was naked, and I hid myself"* (Genesis 3:10). Here, when sin entered the Earth, we have the first use of the word "I" in the Bible. Sin makes us focus on ourselves, including our shortcomings. On the other hand, when God's Spirit is living within us, we focus on our righteousness. Therefore, the soul is self-conscious. As soon as Adam recognized that he was living absent of God's Spirit, he became self-centered. He went from being godly and secure to insecure because his soul was impure, and his self-image was instantly clouded. Unworthiness became his burden, and self-hatred became his reality.

I'm so grateful that God the Father had another plan already in place:

> "And the Lord God said unto the serpent,
>   'Because thou hast done this, thou art cursed
>   above all cattle and above every beast of the
>   field; upon thy belly shalt thou go, and dust
>   shall thou eat all the days of thy life, and I will
>   put enmity between thee and the woman, and
>   between thy seed and her seed; it shall bruise
>   thy head, and thou shalt bruise thy heel."
>
> — GENESIS 3:14-15

Who is the seed of the woman? It's Jesus Christ, the Son of God. God the Father sent Jesus to pay the penalty for sin and to be the sin-offering for all humankind. When Jesus came to the Earth, He walked the Earth sinlessly for 33 years, went to the cross, and laid down His life for the sins of all people.

Next, His Spirit and soul went to hell for three days. While there, He took the keys to death, hell, and the grave (Revelations 1:18). When He resurrected from the dead, He got up with all power in His hands (Matthew 28:18). From there He breathed on His disciples and said to them, *"Receive ye the Holy Ghost"* (John 20:22). For the first time in history, humankind was qualified and ready for the Spirit of God to come back and live within humankind again.

Before this, if God wanted to work through a person, the Spirit of God had to come upon him. That's why the Spirit of God had to come upon Abraham, Isaac, Jacob, Joseph, Moses, Joshua, Sampson, David, Isaiah, Jeremiah, Ezekiel, Daniel, and all the other Old Testament patriarchs.

Jesus coming to the Earth was not only so the Spirit of God could live inside a man again but also so all humankind could be free from any demonic bondage that Satan could wield. That's why Jesus said at the beginning of his earthly ministry, *"The Spirit of the Lord God is upon me because He hath anointed me to preach the gospel unto the poor; He hath sent me to heal the broken-hearted, to preach deliverance to the captives, and to recover sight to the blind, to set at liberty they who are bruised, to preach the acceptable year of the Lord"* (Luke 4:18-19).

Because of Jesus, the Spirit of God can live in you and come upon you to heal your broken heart and to set you free from an ungodly soul tie. You can't do this on your own. You need Jesus.

Now it's time to learn what a soul tie is.

CHAPTER 4
WHAT IS A SOUL TIE?

AT THE TENDER age of 12, I was one of the best-looking young men in the entire sixth-grade class. Therefore, I felt entitled to have the prettiest girlfriend that the sixth grade—or even the seventh grade—had to offer.

Eventually, I got the opportunity to choose the prettiest girl in our class. It wasn't unusual for us to talk on the phone for three or four hours at a time. Sometimes we talked into the early morning hours, knowing that we had to be at school in just a few hours.

I walked her from one class to the next, carrying her books and backpack, common courtesy for the young fellas in those days. It was our way as "young lions" to "mark our territory" around the school.

The first time we kissed, she looked at me and said, "I think you're my soulmate." We held hands often, kissed regularly, and—even at that young age—we engaged in sexual intimacy whenever we got the chance. I know that's extremely young, but when you grow up in the ghetto, in a dysfunctional home, in ignorance, and you lack godly models, it is normal to try to live as the grown-ups around you do.

My junior-high-school sweetheart and I thought we were soul-mates, but we were creating a soul tie, which is the binding, knitting, and cleaving together of two souls. The first soul tie we see in the Bible was created in Genesis 2:23-24: *"And Adam said, 'This is now bone of my bones, and flesh of my flesh; she shall be called "woman," because she was taken from man. Therefore, shall a man leave his father and his mother and shall cleave unto his wife, and they shall be one flesh.'"*

The word "cleave" in the Hebrew language means "attaching oneself to another, to follow hard after and to join completely as one with another." When God the Father created the first man (i.e., Adam) and the first woman (i.e., Eve), his purpose for their marriage was for both Adam and Eve to cleave, to be joined completely as one (i.e., spirit, soul, and body). Therefore, God the Father was the Creator of soul ties. In the beginning, God put the cleaving element into marriage because it was never in His divine plan for spouses to divorce.

Biblically, we see the first soul tie was created in a perfect world with two perfect people who had not sinned. The next reference we see in the Bible as it relates to a soul tie is in Genesis 34:2-3: *"And when Shechem, the son of Hamor the Hivite, Prince of the Country, saw her, he took her and lay with her and defiled her, and his soul clave unto Dinah, the daughter of Jacob, and he loved the damsel and spake kindly unto the damsel."*

In this story, Hamor raped Dinah, and his soul "followed hard" after Dinah—he fell in love with her because his soul cleaved to her. In this situation, it wasn't a godly soul tie; rather, it was an ungodly soul tie.

The next reference to a soul tie in the Scriptures can be seen in the story of Ruth. Naomi, Ruth's mother-in-law, had two daughters-in-law who both had lost their husbands, Naomi's sons. Naomi was returning to her homeland and released her two daughters-in-law to return to their fathers' homes and create new lives for their futures.

Naomi spoke to her daughters-in-law, Ruth and Orpah: *"'For it grieveth me much for your sakes that the hand of the* LORD *is gone out against me,' and they* [Ruth and Orpah] *lifted up their voice and wept again, and Orpah kissed her mother-in-law* [insinuating that she was leaving], *but Ruth clave* [attached oneself to another] *unto* [Naomi]" (Ruth 1:13-14). Ruth stayed with Naomi because her soul was tied to her mother-in-law. If you know the story, then you're aware of why God blessed Ruth with a new husband; it was because she stayed close and faithful to her mother-in-law and took care of her in her old age. If her soul wouldn't have cleaved (i.e., been tied to Naomi), then she wouldn't have gone to Naomi's homeland, found a new husband, and taken care of Naomi.

Our working definition of a soul tie is *the binding, knitting, and cleaving together of two souls.*

Let's see how the language changes in the story of Joseph. We pick up when the sons of Jacob went to Egypt to buy corn during a famine. To their surprise, their brother Joseph, whom they had thrown into a pit and sold into slavery many years prior, was Prime Minister of Egypt, and he was playing a trick on them to see if his younger brother, Benjamin, was still alive.

Joseph had told the brothers to return to Israel and bring back his brother Benjamin. If they did not, he would not sell them any more food. Judah said unto Joseph in Genesis, *"Now, therefore when I come to thy servant my father, and the lad be not with us, seeing that his life is bound up in the lad's life, it shall come to pass when he seeth that the lad is not with us, that he will die"* (Genesis 44:30-31). Jacob's entire life was bound up in Benjamin's life is to say that Jacob's soul was bound to his son's—he had a soul tie.

In the story of David and Jonathan, David had just defeated Goliath. Saul took David to be his armor-bearer. Because the plan of God was in place to take the kingdom of Israel from Saul and give it to David, in God's sovereignty, he allowed the souls of Jonathan and David to be knitted together: *"And it came to pass when David had made an end of speaking unto Saul, that the soul of Jonathan was knit with the soul of David, and Jonathan loved David as his own soul"* (1 Samuel 18:1). The word "knit" in Hebrew means "to tie, bind, or be woven together." God was the orchestrator of the soul knitting between David and Jonathan.

Finally, in 1 Kings, we see the downfall of King Solomon, the son of David:

> "But King Solomon loved many strange women,
>   together with the daughter of Pharaoh,
>   women of the Moabites, Ammonites,
>   Edomites, Zidonians, and Hittites, of the
>   nations concerning which the LORD said unto
>   the children of Israel, 'Ye shall not go into
>   them; neither shall they come in unto you, for
>   surely they will turn away your heart after
>   their gods; Solomon clave unto these in love.'"
>
> — 1 KINGS 11:1–2

One thing I've learned about life and relationships is that when God is ready to elevate your life, he connects you with the right person. On the other hand, when the enemy wants to take you down, he connects you with the wrong person. The purpose of any relational connection is either to add value to you or to take value from you.

The more Solomon cleaved to those strange and foreign women, the more his heart grew cold toward the true and living God. It took a while, but eventually, Solomon's heart turned away from God completely, and his life didn't end well.

I took the time to show you these scriptures to make this point: Though the Bible doesn't use the term "soul tie," the concept that the soul can bond, knit, or cleave to something, thereby resulting in your soul being tied to someone or something, is clear in the scriptures.

If you don't like the term *soul tie*, you could call it a *covenant connection* because as soon as you allow your soul to make a covenant or vow with something or someone, you've formed a connection.

According to Scripture, soul ties come from two sources: either godly soul ties or ungodly soul ties. God the Father is the Creator and the originator of all things, which is why he created soul ties in marriage. You can't control the family you were born into, but you are tied to your family members. There are friendships and partnerships with which God connects you for his purpose. Your soul can get tied to your friend or partner. These are soul ties that come from God.

On the other hand, because God the Father is the Creator and originator of all things, the adversary (Satan, the enemy) is always looking for opportunities to duplicate and pervert whatever God the Father creates. Therefore, ungodly soul ties come from the enemy.

The term *soul tie* is one of the most divisive, misunderstood, and confusing terms in the church because it's wrongly associated with having a demonic spirit. But soul ties and demonic spirits are not the same, even though demonic spirits have a soul.

Jesus said, *"When the unclean spirit is gone from a man, he walketh through dry places, seeking rest, and findeth none"* (Matthew 12:43). This means if a spirit is looking for something, then he's thinking. Remember the functions of the soul: the mind (i.e., the thinker), the will (i.e., the chooser), the emotions (i.e., the feeler), the memory (i.e., the replayer of thoughts, feelings, actions, and scenes), the imagination (i.e., the previewer of potential scenes, visions, and possibilities), and the personality (i.e., the character, behavior, mood, and consistent attitude). According to this verse, an unclean spirit "seeks rest." The word "rest" means "to find comfort and relief, to be in a state of peace." If comfort, release, and peace are associated with rest, then this informs us how rest relates to our emotions.

In Matthew 12:44 the idea continues: *"I will return into my house from whence I came out, and when he has come, he findeth it empty, swept, and garnished."* When the demonic spirit says, "I will return," we see how the will and the memory of the spirit are in operation. In an act of his will, he believes he can go back into a body he had previously occupied. To believe he could go back means he could remember or recall how he had been there previously.

I'm not saying that soul ties and demonic spirits are the same, but I am saying that demonic spirits are disembodied spirits that have a soul, and they are looking for any type of body to get inside, whether it's human or animal.

When Adam ate from the Tree of the Knowledge of Good and Evil in Genesis 3, he rebelled against God; the Spirit of God left Adam. Also, Adam passed his dominion to Satan, and sin entered the Earth. At that point, everything God created to be holy, Satan turned unholy—even the binding, knitting, and cleaving of two souls.

HOW SOUL TIES ARE CREATED

Whether they are godly or ungodly, soul ties are created by way of sexual intercourse (e.g., in marriage, same-sex activity, or fornication), emotional attachments, or vows and promises made in a covenant agreement. In marriage, two become one via a covenant agreement, emotional attachment, and sexual intercourse. In Hebrew culture, the word "covenant" means "a permanent arrangement." That's why God puts two people together in a marriage that is designed to be permanent (Mark 10:7-9).

In the eyes of God, marriage isn't just a contract. The word "contract" means "a binding agreement." Your words hold you to whatever you agreed to in the contract. A contract can be broken easier than a covenant. A contract is typically temporary, but a covenant is designed to be permanent. A contract is a natural agreement, but a covenant is a spiritual agreement. A contract is a one-time commitment that may be broken, but a covenant is a long-term guarantee.

Next, you have an emotional attachment. This is when two people are willing to be 100% vulnerable by allowing all their emotions to become one with the emotions of their spouse, friend, or partner. It's an act of will when you allow your emotions to attach to another person early in a relationship.

Following the emotional attachment is a vow and a promise. A vow dedicates yourself to someone or something, even to a deity. A promise is a declaration or an assurance that you will do a particular thing. You make a vow by what you say to a person, but you make a promise by what you say to yourself. A lot of times people make vows outwardly, but they never make a promise inwardly. That's why you can be in love with someone who's not in love with you. When you vow or promise to connect yourself to something or someone, you're allowing yourself to be tied spiritually and emotionally.

Last is confirmation, which is the action of making a union complete by way of sexual intercourse. The two become one by way of spirit, soul, and body under either a godly instruction (marriage) or an ungodly instruction (sexual relationship).

Let's look at what the Bible says when you create a soul tie in an ungodly way:

> "Don't you know that your bodies belong to
> Christ as His body parts? Should one presume
> to take the members of Christ's body and
> make them into members of a harlot? Abso-
> lutely not! Aren't you aware of the fact that
> when anyone sleeps with a prostitute, he
> becomes a part of her, and she becomes a part
> of him? For it has been declared, the two
> become one single body, but the one who joins
> himself unto the lord is mingled into one spirit
> with Him. This is why you must keep running
> away from sexual immorality, for every other

sin a person commits is external to the body,
but immorality involves sinning against your
own body. Have you forgotten that your body
is now the Sacred Temple of the Spirit of Holi-
ness who lives inside you? You don't belong to
yourself any longer, for the gift of God, the
Holy Spirit, lives inside your sanctuary. You
were God's expensive purchase, paid for with
tears of blood. So, by all means, then, use your
body to bring glory to God."

— 1 CORINTHIANS 6:15-21 (TPT)

The writer, the apostle Paul, is explaining how our physical
bodies are no longer our own. If you're a Christian, he wants
you to value the fact that your body belongs to Jesus Christ.
Don't forget, when a person accepts Jesus as her personal Lord
and Savior, the Holy Spirit, which is the Spirit of Christ (1 Peter
1:11), and the Spirit of the Father (Matthew 10:20) join with
your spirit and becomes one with your spirit.

Therefore, He's not only your Savior but also your Lord. So, if
He's your Lord, then He owns you, and your body becomes
His body. Therefore, the Bible says that you are the body of
Christ (1 Corinthians 12:12-13). According to Verse 15, anytime
a Christian has sex outside marriage, it's fornication, and the
Christian becomes one with the harlot (i.e., the prostitute).
Therefore, Paul is warning us of the danger of sex outside
marriage when he says, *"Aren't you aware of the fact that when a
person sleeps with a prostitute, he becomes a part of her, and she
becomes a part of him? For it has been declared, the two become a
single body"* (1 Corinthians 6:16).

Today, fornication is the norm, as are live-in relationships and common-law marriages. As you can see, these are against what the Word of God says about the body of Christ because they create ungodly, unhealthy soul ties. 1 Corinthians 6:17 reads, *"But he that is joined unto the Lord is one spirit."* The next verse states why we must run away from sexual immorality: *"Flee fornication. Every sin that a man doeth is without the body, but he that committeth fornication sinneth against his own body"* (1 Corinthians 6:18).

FOUR TYPES OF LOVE

Going back to the story of my sixth-grade girlfriend, we thought we were in love, and we assumed that we were each other's soulmate, simply because we didn't have a correct or godly revelation about love. We confused love with lust. Anytime you say the word "love," know that there are four distinct types of love. The first type of love is "agape," which is the unconditional love of God that is displayed through Jesus in all four of the Gospels. His love for us isn't based on what we do (i.e., our performance); it's based on who we are. Anytime love is based on who you are, there will never be any conditions tied to it.

Many stories in the Bible prove the unconditional love of God (i.e., agape). For one, the story of the prodigal son is found in Luke 15:11-32. Two sons and a father are the characters in this story. One day, the younger son told the father to give him his part of the inheritance that would be his upon his father's death. He wanted his inheritance immediately. He was really saying to his father, "I wish you were dead." A godly soul tie existed between this father and son; therefore, the father didn't want anything to come between their love, so he granted his son's wish.

The younger son packed up his possessions, moved to another country, and wasted his inheritance on riotous living. When you study the term "riotous living," one definition you may find is a playboy lifestyle, which is the idea of a man having multiple sex partners, whom he supports financially.

Once the younger son spent all his inheritance, famine hit the land, and he was stuck in extreme poverty. To find work to support himself, he became a citizen of the country, so he could be legally employed. As soon as the younger son found a job, his employer sent him to feed swine in the fields. Things got worse for the younger son, and he was tempted to eat the swine's food because he was in such a crisis. Even worse—it was against his culture and his royal position to work in a swine field.

As soon as the pressure piled up, and he came to his senses, a thought came to him: *"How many hired servants of my father have bread enough to spare, while I'm dying of starvation? I will arise and go to my father, and I will say to my father, 'Father, I have sinned against Heaven and before thee and am no more worthy to be called "thy son," make me as one of thy hired servants.'"*

The younger son quit his job and went back to his own country. As soon as he got within sight of his home, his father saw him, had compassion, ran to him, threw his arms around him, and kissed him! Can you see the (agape) unconditional love the father had for his son? Even though his son had acted like an illegitimate child, the father was full of forgiveness and was waiting on the son to come home.

After the hugs and kisses, the younger son started repenting and trying to undervalue his position as his father's child. The father never agreed with the younger son when he tried to convince him that he wasn't worthy to be called his son. The father called to his servants. "Bring the best robe and place it on him, put the ring on his finger, and shoes on his feet."

In biblical times, the robe represented the younger son's righteousness. When the father put the robe on the younger son, it was letting everyone know that the younger son was fully back in alignment and standing with his father. The ring represented authority. So, when the father put the ring on the younger son's hand, it proved that his authority was restored. Finally, the shoes represented his rights as a son. As soon as the father put the shoes on his son's feet, everyone knew that his rights as a son had been fully restored.

The message the father's actions conveyed to his son, family, and community was that nothing could break the agape love he had for his son. The father's love was not based on the son's behavior; rather, it was based on his position as a son.

It's amazing that because the son came home destitute and in rags, he was unable to reestablish his authority or righteousness for his rights; the father had to do it for him. The father didn't make the son go through a process of rebuilding trust to ensure that he wouldn't do this again. The father's love is so unconditional that he reestablished his son as soon as he saw him. Please know that God the Father will reestablish you as soon as you repent from an ungodly soul tie.

The second type of love is "phileo." It's a friendship bond and love. This is the type of bond David and Jonathan had, which we learned about in 1 Samuel 18. The Bible says that Jonathan loved David as his own soul. Even though Jonathan was supposed to inherit the throne as the next king of Israel, Jonathan knew that God anointed David to be king, so he transferred his right of kingship over to David.

God placed phileo love in the heart of Jonathan, which resulted in a godly soul tie. That's why Jonathan would not allow envy, jealousy, or hate to motivate him to help his father Saul kill David. Instead, he protected David from his father and made a covenant with his friend to ensure that all his family members would have favor with David on the day he would become king. They had a brotherly love that was undeniable, unbreakable, and untouchable.

The third type of love is *storgeo*. This is a family bond, an empathetic bond, and overall love for people. This is the type of love people naturally have for their families (or a friend who feels like family). It's the love Ruth had for Naomi. The empathetic bond would not allow her to sever the soul tie she had developed with her mother-in-law.

The final type of love is "eros." This is intense, passionate love that is highly sensual—and even intoxicating. It describes strong desires, ranging from patriotism to sexual love. It is a love that is desirous of something: craving, lust, passion, or fulfillment. This is the type of love the enemy uses to create ungodly and unhealthy soul ties. This love starts as pure and undefiled because it originates from God the Father, but when our motives are impure, what's pure becomes impure. God incorporated this passionate, lustful, and romantic love into the context of marriage. Eros love is for a married couple to enjoy their sexual life and procreate.

My sixth-grade girlfriend and I had eros love. When we should have been relating to each other through phileo or storgeo love, we took it upon ourselves to create and experience eros love.

Our familial culture insinuated that we didn't love each other if we weren't having sexual intercourse. Therefore, we took it upon ourselves to create love in an unhealthy and ungodly way. We broke up a year later. She was extremely heartbroken, struggled with low self-esteem, and was highly embarrassed because I had taken her innocence. To be honest, I didn't know every thought and feeling that was tormenting her, but I know our sexual relationship had an unhealthy effect on both of us.

I went onto the next girlfriend, and eventually she found another boyfriend. Did we have sexual relationships with our next partners? Absolutely! Guess what? We each created a new soul tie. Think about how many ties a person can accumulate throughout 10, 20, or even 30 years!

What we didn't know was that sexual immorality is a sin. It's demonic, and it created an ungodly soul tie that led to a negative effect for both of us, possibly for the rest of our lives. I'm sure we would have been a lot healthier for our permanent spouses if only we had been taught the truth about the four distinct types of love, and the danger of creating ungodly and unhealthy soul ties.

CHAPTER 5

HOW DO I KNOW IF I'M TIED?

Soul ties, or covenant connections if you prefer, are extremely powerful because they're not just physical connections but spiritual and emotional connections. When the connection is spiritual and emotional, it's something you can feel but not see.

People in America and Western culture have been trained by society to believe a thing only if they can see it—that's materialism. That thinking is directly against the Bible's teaching because the Word of God says, *"We walk by faith, not by sight"* (2 Corinthians 5:7). If you believe the things you see only, you don't believe the spirit world is real because you can't see the spirit world with your physical eyes.

The Bible says clearly, *"Through faith, we understand that the worlds were framed by the Word of God, so that things which are seen were not made of things which do appear"* (Hebrews 11:3). What do you do if you cannot see what you feel? If you believe only the things you see, then you've turned the God of the Universe into a human being. The truth is that what you can't see is 100 times more real than what you can see. That's why soul ties and covenant connections are so powerful; you can't see with your eyes the ties that bind a person to another person or thing, but the person who is bound can feel those bindings.

The following are examples of the ties that bind us:

- **Family Ties:** We all have soul ties of one kind or another. Your soul can be tied to your family members, which is a family soul tie. It is common and normal for your soul to develop a strong bond or a tie with your mother, father, sister, brother, grandparents, aunts, uncles, and especially your child. Family is important because God designed the family unit and gave you the family to be tied to.

- **Friendly Ties:** Your soul can be tied to your friends and associates. If you allow your soul to follow hard after or get attached to a friend or an associate, the connection can turn into a tie. That's why it's normal for two friends to hurt if there is confusion or separation in their relationship.

- **Interpersonal Ties:** Your soul can be tied to your mentor, teacher, coach, or advisor. These are relationships that can form a strong bond as two people work and grow together. Both people will begin to care about the other's mental, emotional, personal, and financial well-being as the relationship grows.

- **Spiritual Ties:** One of the most powerful forms of discipleship takes place by way of spiritual parenting. God places spiritual parents into the lives of young children so that growth and discipleship can develop. The apostle Paul was a spiritual father to Timothy, Priscilla, Aquila, Titus, and a host of others. *"For though you might have 10,000 instructors in Christ, yet you do not* *have many fathers; for in Christ Jesus, I have begotten you through the gospel"* (1 Corinthians 4:15 [NKJV]). You can tell by the way that the apostle Paul opens his letters in 1 and 2 Timothy that the two men's souls were tied.

- **Past-Life Ties:** Your soul can be tied to your past life, a nickname, an old reputation, or an ungodly belief system that you once held. This is how the enemy keeps a person in bondage mentally—even though God the Father has set them free spiritually. When I gave my life to God and Christ completely back in November 2006, the best thing that happened to me at that time was that I received a disciplinary transfer from the Atlanta prison camp to FCI Big Spring in Big Spring, Texas. In the natural, most people would view this as negative, but through this event, I had the opportunity to sever the ungodly soul ties I had with my past life, former nickname, old reputation, and the ungodly belief system I had developed through my former poverty mindset.

As soon as I walked onto the prison yard, the first person I met asked me where I was from, and what my name was. Instantly, I heard the Spirit of God say in my heart, *"You don't have to live a lie for another day. You are a new creation in Christ; you have a new future, and you're beginning a new life. Therefore, it's time to change your name. Your name is not Butch anymore; your name is James. Tell him your real name."*

And I did. I told people that I go by James. Up until that moment, I had been living by the nickname "Butch." But Butch had led me to receive an eight-year federal prison sentence, hurting a lot of people in the past, and developing a selfish and ungodly mindset.

The beautiful thing about being at FCI Big Spring was that not one person there knew of me or my past. Therefore, when I told people my name was James, that's what they called me. I didn't have to be reminded of or respond to that past nickname that helped me build a superficial identity. God was giving me a fresh start, and it was up to me to detach myself from that old, ungodly identity. That's why the Bible says, *"Therefore, if anyone is in Christ, he is a new creation; old things have passed away; behold, all things have become new"* (2 Corinthians 5:17 [NKJV]). If you can't sever or detach your soul from a negative past, then you will only have an ungodly future.

THE THREE LEVELS OF A SOUL TIE

There are three levels of soul ties. The first is the heavy soul tie. Second, a moderate soul tie, and last, a light soul tie.

A heavy soul tie makes you feel like you can't live without that person or thing you're bound to. I can remember when I couldn't sleep or eat because Jessica, with whom I had a heavy soul tie, had left me while I was in prison. It's an everyday fight to loosen its heaviness. A heavy soul tie will cause you to want to lay down and die because the pain seems unbearable. When you think about your mate not reconnecting with you, a spirit of terror can pierce your heart.

The moderate tie will often play tricks on you if your mind isn't made up. This level of soul tie will take you on a roller-coaster ride for years if you allow it. One day, you'll feel like you're ready to move forward, but the next day, you'll feel like your life is incomplete without your ex. A moderate soul tie will cause you to appear unstable, hypocritical, and emotionally weak. If you don't have self-control, then a moderate soul tie will make you double-minded.

You feel the light soul tie, but you can move forward. You know that you're still tied, but you can function and live with it. Its control is minimal, and every day you get better and better. When the tie feels light, this is when you know you're winning and eventually you'll be victorious.

SEVEN SIGNS THAT INDICATE YOU'RE TIED

Anytime I find myself in a conversation about soul ties, one of the most frequently asked questions I get is, "How do I know if I have an ungodly or unhealthy soul tie?"

As it pertains to past relationships, here are seven signs that will let you know if you have an ungodly soul tie:

1. YOU WILLINGLY STARTED YOUR RELATIONSHIP IN DISOBEDIENCE TO GOD'S WORD.

Maybe you're wondering how you can know if you were disobedient. Did you have a gut feeling that something wasn't right? Did your friends or family members try to influence you not to connect with this person? What did your mom and dad say when they found out you were in a relationship with this person?

Believers in Christ should always consider the most essential element before starting an intimate relationship that they hope will lead to marriage: Does God approve of this relationship? The Bible says, *"Trust in the Lord with all thine heart; lean not unto thine own understanding. In all thy ways, acknowledge Him, and He shall direct thy path"* (Proverbs 3:5-6). Christians' lives are not our own. We've been bought with a price. Therefore, we don't have the liberty to make life-altering decisions without the council of God. The choice of whom you marry or develop a soul tie with can either push you toward your God-given destiny or into early destruction.

A biblical example to help you understand this is found in Judges 13. Read the entire story of Samson. God purposed Samson to deliver God's chosen people out of the hand of the enemy (the Philistines). God gifted Samson with supernatural strength. Anytime Samson found himself fighting the Philistines, the Spirit of God came upon him, and he destroyed the Philistines with his bare hands.

On one occasion, Samson destroyed 1000 men with only a jawbone of a donkey. Even though Samson was physically strong, he was emotionally weak when it came to women. One of the most important instructions God gave to Samson was that he was not to take any woman outside of his people (Judges 14:3). Samson rebelled not just one time but three times.

The Philistines fought Samson on many occasions, but they couldn't defeat him—until they discovered where his strength came from. So, instead of continuing to fight Samson and losing, they figured out they needed to identify his weakness, so they could lessen his strength. They knew Samson would take the bait and go for a beautiful Philistine woman; therefore, they made a deal with Delilah to help destroy him.

Because Samson was disobedient to the instructions of God, he developed a soul tie with Delilah, a Philistine. Eventually, Delilah led Samson straight into the Philistine's trap.

I've always wondered why human beings are so comfortable operating in disobedience to God's instruction when it comes to relationships. One day I had a thought that I believe came from the Spirit of God: *Attraction doesn't have to equate to selection, but it does because of desperation.*

You should never feel pressured to select someone just because you are attracted to that person. Any attraction that pushes you to make a selection without God's instruction will lead to destruction because if you select them without God's approval, you must have everything you need to fix the relationship if it breaks.

Most people don't understand that you attract who you are, but God gives you instructions to make a selection based on where you're going. God knows the direction in which He wants your life to go; therefore, He would recommend that you choose with your future in mind. On the other hand, desperation will push you to choose with your present or past in mind. When desperation causes you to disobey, you will find yourself connected to an ungodly soul tie.

2. YOU MAKE EXCUSES FOR THEIR ABUSE.

If you're in a relationship in which your partner continually cheats on you, physically and/or verbally abuses you, and/or takes advantage of you, but you make excuses for them when others point out the problem to you, that's a strong indication that you have an ungodly soul tie.

The purpose of a relationship is for two people to come together and bring out the best in each other. They are to build each other up, not tear each other down. It's not normal to allow constant verbal, mental, financial, or physical abuse. Maybe you allow it because you're afraid of being alone, or maybe you tolerate it because the abuser has made you believe that nobody else will want you. Whatever the reason you tolerate the abuse and excuse the behavior, it's a soul tie.

Don't forget that anything you tolerate will dominate you. So, if you tolerate cheating, then cheating will dominate you. If you tolerate physical, mental, emotional, or verbal abuse, then it will dominate you. Making an excuse for your abuser is not normal; it's dysfunctional. God didn't create relationships to function in abuse. Allowing it and excusing it goes against the purpose of which God intended relationships to be. That, my friend, is dysfunctional.

Why would you make excuses for a person who is destroying you? One reason is that your soul is tied heavily to the person.

3. EVERY TIME YOU GO BACK TO THE ABUSER, THE RELATIONSHIP GETS WORSE.

For example, at some point in the relationship, the two of you continue arguing, disagreeing, and not being on the same page. It causes you to recognize the relationship isn't adding value to you, or maybe you two are not cohesive enough to grow. So finally, you build up the courage to walk away.

Sometime later, you feel lonely and want to speak to your ex to see if you two can start over. Because your partner missed you too, you both agree to give the relationship another shot. Months, or weeks, later, the arguing and disagreeing escalate. That's when you recognize again that you two haven't matured enough to rebuild what you once tore down.

So, mutually, you call it quits again. As time progresses, both of you feel like you can't make it without each other. So, you come back to try to work it out. Months later, you discover that your mate is cheating on you. To prove to the competition that you will be the one who ends up with the prize, you fight for the relationship by forgiving them and staying together.

A year later, your mate is still cheating. Once again, you break up and go your separate ways. Deep in your heart, you know it's not over. So, you rekindle the relationship—although the dysfunction is still present. A few months pass. So much hurt and disrespect has taken place in the relationship; therefore, neither one of you can control your temper. It's no longer just verbal fights, but it's gotten worse; you two are having physical altercations…often.

It's clear that you two are not good for each other, but you still feel like you can't live without each other. Therefore, for the next several years, you stay connected, on and off. The scariest part about your relationship is that every time you break up and get back together, your dysfunction and abuse intensify. When things start getting rocky, your mindset is, *"I've got to cheat on them before they cheat on me,"* or, *"I have to abuse them before they abuse me."*

The trust and love are long gone. The only thing keeping you two together is lust and trauma. Truth be told, you two will spend the future in an abusive and toxic relationship because you believe that you don't have any power to break free from the connection; it feels so strong. The one principle you didn't learn was: "never make a decision based on your feelings, anytime your feelings go against your godly future." That's why you have an unhealthy and ungodly soul tie.

4. YOU ARE MENTALLY CONSUMED WITH CERTAIN QUESTIONS BUT YOU TWO ARE NOT TOGETHER.

You may often find yourself asking, *"What are they doing? Are they okay? Do they miss me? Will we ever get back together? Are they thinking about me like I'm thinking about them?"*

If you two have broken up, separated, divorced, or been apart for six months, a year, two years, or longer, and these questions continue to permeate your mind, then you have a soul tie. Though you are delivered from the person physically, you're not free mentally, spiritually, or emotionally. This is the major difference between deliverance and freedom from ungodly soul ties.

Deliverance is established when you break up or separate from this person, and you do not see each other regularly, but freedom is when the thoughts, memories, and visions about that person leave your mind, and there is zero effect on you. Deliverance is physical separation, while freedom is emotional and internal liberation. When your thoughts are consumed with this other person, when you can't focus, move forward, or remain consistent in growth and maturity, you are still tied to them. This person is still living inside your mind rent-free. If this is happening to you, then you may be delivered from them, but you are not free.

If you're thinking about this person constantly, then you may make social-media posts about them, hoping and praying that they will see them. You may want their attention and approval and hope they send you a DM.

It gets dangerous when you value this person's opinion and approval over God's. If you are consumed with thinking about them, then it is because you don't believe you can control your thoughts. If you want to break free, then you must receive the conviction of this truth: Just because thoughts of them cross your mind doesn't mean you have to feed into those thoughts. You have control over what you give your attention to. If you don't grasp this truth, then you'll remain in bondage to these uncontrolled thoughts for the rest of your life. Anytime God performs an act of liberation, He starts in your spirit. After He frees your spirit, then He will partner with you and teach you how to free your mind.

Most Christians don't live victorious lives because although they are free spiritually, they're in bondage mentally. They are going to Heaven, but they are living in hell right here on Earth. Complete freedom from an ungodly soul tie is mental and emotional freedom. Gaining freedom is a battle, but victory is guaranteed. Therefore, mentally you have to learn to fight from a position *of* victory and not *for* victory.

5. YOU HAVE SEVERAL DREAMS ABOUT SOMEONE YOU'VE BEEN SEXUALLY INTIMATE WITH, EVEN THOUGH YOU'RE NOT IN A RELATIONSHIP ANYMORE.

Remember that there are light soul ties, moderate soul ties, and heavy soul ties. Depending on which one you are wrestling with will determine what you do on the morning you wake up after the dream.

After you have a sex dream about a person, and you try to rekindle the relationship or pursue sex with that person, you're struggling with a heavy-to-moderate soul tie. If you want to contact that person, but you're fighting with yourself not to call or reach out, then you still have a moderate-to-light soul tie.

Your dreams have the ability to show you what's going on in your heart. If this person is still living in your heart, then the consistency of your dreams will let you know the severity of the tie. Therefore, don't discount your dreams; they are showing you what type of soul tie you still have to this person.

6. YOU START TALKING, THINKING, ACTING, AND LIVING LIKE THAT PERSON.

This is the effect of what the Bible says: *"The two shall become one flesh"* (Genesis 2:24). Anytime you join life with a person, especially if you become sexually intimate, you make a strong emotional connection. You should expect that person's ways, habits, and lifestyle to become a part of you.

This is both a positive and negative aspect. When I met my wife in 2014, I was single and living a bachelor's lifestyle. The first time I stepped into her condo, I said to myself, *"This house is spotless!"* It was so clean; you could eat off the floor. My apartment wasn't nasty, but no one could accuse me of being a clean freak.

We got married in 2016. Can you guess what our #1 disagreement has always been? My lack of cleanliness, according to her standards. My lifelong habit of coming into a house, taking off my shoes, and leaving them there until I put them on the next day drives my wife crazy! Not to mention, every now and then, I'll leave my clothes on the couch or a dirty cup in the sink. If she comes home from work to find a less-than-spotless house, then she sees that as I'm disrespecting her. Cleanliness means so much to her; therefore, she feels that it should mean the same to me.

She says, "Listen, sir, cleanliness means a lot to me. When it comes to this area of our marriage, I'm not coming down to where you are; you're going to have to come up to where I am, and that's final!"

Marriage has taught me two principles. The first principle is that by becoming one with a person, you're either going to take on your mate's weakness, or their strength. Therefore, you'll have to either come up to where they are, or you'll bring them down to where you are. In my situation, my wife, Tiffaney, is strongest when it comes to cleanliness, so maturity presses me to come up to where she is. If I let immaturity reign, then I would drag her down to where I am.

Marriage is for the mature because only the immature will embrace laziness and allow weakness to block the peace of God from reigning over your relationship. Therefore, I decided to embrace the challenge of becoming a "neat freak." Now that we have a gorgeous new home, I want to keep it clean so that when people walk through the door, they feel like it's a model home. Let's say that I've made some significant adjustments to my cleanliness!

The second principle I learned is that if it matters to your spouse, then it must also matter to you. You'll never experience true intimacy in a marriage or relationship if you don't embrace this principle. When what matters to your mate also matters to you, only then can you allow all of them to become one with you. That's what it means when the Bible says the two have become one. The bonding, knitting, and cleaving of your souls will strengthen. When you take on their ways, style, attractions, and appetites, then you have a soul tie.

7. YOU RECOGNIZE THAT THE RELATIONSHIP IS TOXIC, MISERABLE, AND UNFRUITFUL, BUT YOU STAY IN IT.

Nobody in their right mind wants to remain connected to someone whom they know isn't adding value to them or doesn't want to be with them.

It's toxic to be miserable and feel as if there's nothing you can do about it. It's unhealthy to know your relationship is sinking into destruction but you feel compelled to go down with the ship. When others tell you that your relationship is horrible, it's sad and embarrassing that you feel like you must accept it for what it is.

To solve a problem, you must first identify the problem. Hopefully, these seven indicators of soul ties have helped you figure out if you're wrestling with an ungodly soul tie.

PART TWO
SIX SECRETS OF SOUL TIES

CHAPTER 6

SECRET #1—IGNORANCE OR DENIAL

JESUS MADE a powerful statement that has been a passkey I've used to free myself from ungodly soul ties and help others break free from all types of bondage, including unhealthy and ungodly soul ties. Jesus said, *"If ye continue in My Word, then ye are My disciples; indeed, and ye shall know the truth, and the truth shall make you free"* (John 8:31-32).

We must meet a condition if we want to be Jesus' disciples: We must continue in His Word. This is true not only if we want to be His disciples but also to obtain spiritual freedom. According to Jesus, we must continue in His Word. These verses reveal that the more of Jesus' Word we keep, the more freedom we will receive. If spiritual, mental, and emotional freedom is your pursuit, then continue reading, practicing, meditating, living, and becoming the Word of God. At that point, you will know the truth, and the truth will make you free.

Now, the greatest question of all time arises: "What is truth?" I would love to use the illustration that the great Dr. Myles Munroe used in his book, *the Spirit of Leadership*: *"Truth is orig-*

inal information."[1] Therefore, original information can only come from the manufacturer of a product. So, if God is the manufacturer, and we are the products, then the only One who has the original information about us is God.

Since Jesus came into the world 100% God and 100% man, He defeated death, hell, and the grave when He lived a sinless life, was crucified on the cross, died, was buried, and resurrected Himself from the dead. He earned the right and paid the price to be the Manufacturer of Life and all humankind. He said, *"I am the Way, the Truth, and the Life; no man cometh unto the Father but by Me"* (John 14:6). Paul said, *"Therefore, God also has highly exalted Him [Jesus] and given Him the name which is above every name, that at the name of Jesus, every knee should bow, of those in Heaven and of those on Earth and of those under the Earth, and that every tongue shall confess that Jesus Christ is Lord, to the glory of God the Father"* (Philippians 2:9-11 [NKJV]).

Now that we understand this truth and agree that truth is original information, which is Jesus, this verse tells us that before being introduced to the Word of God, we were not free but in bondage. Not knowing his Word means living by our own, or someone else's, word and standard.

Jesus said as he prayed to God the Father, *"Sanctify them through Thy Truth; Thy Word is Truth"* (John 17:17). According to John 8:31-32, as soon as a person accepts, believes, and receives God's Word, the Word (i.e., truth) ushers us into a new level of spiritual freedom. So, if truth (i.e., God's Word) sets us free, then lies (i.e., untruth) will keep us in bondage. Let's get this conviction settled in our hearts. Jesus wants us to be free, but Satan (i.e., the enemy) wants us to be in bondage.

Please keep in mind this definition for the word "bondage:" "the condition of not being liberated or free because you are strongly influenced by someone or something." Bondage refers to a position of slavery but it's not physical; instead, it's mental, spiritual, and emotional.

The most dangerous thing about relational bondage is that you can accept it both consciously and subconsciously. Jesus said, *"Thy Word is Truth"* (John 17:17), and He called Satan *"the father of lies"* (John 8:44). Jesus' Word leads you to truth and freedom, but Satan's words lead you to lies and bondage. The only way Satan can lead you into bondage or trap you in bondage is for you to believe, accept, receive, and agree with his lies.

I titled this book *The Secret of the Soul Tie* because Satan knows that if you don't uncover his lies, you'll remain tied to hurt, dysfunction, toxicity, powerlessness, fear, guilt, condemnation, shame, pain, and brokenness, all of which come from ungodly and unhealthy soul ties. As soon as you uncover Satan's lies, you can untangle that tie. The lie must die.

The word "secret" means "not known or seen; not meant to be known or seen by others; something that is kept or meant to be kept unknown or unseen by others." As my wife and I have counseled, advised, and discipled countless people through the process of severing ungodly and unhealthy soul ties, the Holy Spirit has revealed to us some of Satan's most common secrets, which he uses to keep believers and nonbelievers tied. In this section of the book, we will expose his secrets, so you can learn and apply the truth, thus defeating him.

The most common and powerful secret Satan wants you to believe can be boiled down to this: soul ties are nonexistent. In other words, an ungodly soul tie does not want you to know it exists. Why doesn't the enemy want you to know ungodly soul ties exist? Because if you don't know an ungodly or unhealthy soul tie exists, you'll allow it to oppress you.

Anytime ungodly soul ties oppress you because you are ignorant of their existence, your mind will accept this oppression as normal. "Oppression" is "to feel overpowered, constrained, entangled, or powerless to cruel, unreasonable, and rigorous government."[4] Whenever demonic oppression is present in your life because of an ungodly or unhealthy soul tie, your connection to that person makes you powerless or constrained against your will. It feels as if there's nothing you can do to overcome the weight and burden of the oppression. If we are ignorant to the enemy's use of ungodly soul ties or ungodly covenant connections to oppress us, then we will live defeated lives. The Bible says, *"For we are not ignorant of* [Satan's] *devices"* (2 Corinthians 2:11). We must understand the enemy's tricks, traps, and schemes, and we must examine how he uses his key weapons to steal, kill, and destroy our lives.

What better or easier way for him to destroy your life than to use the closest person to you, the one with whom you're in covenant? If you don't believe soul ties are real, then you're a candidate for destruction. God said through the mouth of Hosea the prophet, *"My people are destroyed for lack of knowledge; because thou hast rejected knowledge, I will also reject thee, that thou shalt be no priest to Me; seeing thou hast forgotten the law of thy God, I will also forget thy children"* (Hosea 4:6 [NKJV]).

In Chapter 4, I intentionally and unapologetically laid the foundation for the validity and authenticity of soul ties in scripture so that no one would have any excuse to remain ignorant about soul ties or covenant connections. According to Hosea 4:6, the enemy can and will destroy you for lack of knowledge. Ignorance is not a derogatory word; it just means you lack information about a specific thing. We've all been ignorant about something, but just because we are ignorant about something doesn't mean we have to stay ignorant. You're reading this book because you are ready to come out of ignorance about soul ties. You don't want to remain ignorant of soul ties because you don't want to give the enemy the opportunity to use a person whom you're unhealthily tied to against you.

Anytime you see the following three things operating in your mate, friend, sibling, or coworker as it pertains to you, the enemy is trying to gain control over your life. Pay attention to manipulation, intimidation, and domination in your relationships. Whenever any one or more of these elements are present with your spouse, parents, siblings, coaches, coworkers, mentors, or covenant connections, whether they are conscious or subconscious, they are trying to control you to act or live in a way that's beneficial to them, regardless of how it feels to you.

The first sign to alert you to a person seeking control over you is manipulation. The word "manipulation" is defined as "to control or influence a person or a situation cleverly, unfairly, or unscrupulously." Manipulation is an attempt to sway others' emotions to get them to act or feel a certain way. Manipulation will express itself through certain tricks that make you feel uncomfortable, but it will compel you to do what the other person wants you to do. From there, you'll be more likely to give in to the request.

The following are five ways to spot manipulation:

1. The person you're in a relationship with often tries to make you feel guilty.
2. The person you're in a relationship with often tries to trick you into getting their way.
3. The person you're in a relationship with compares you to others to get you to do what they want.

4. The person you're in a relationship with lies to get you to make the choices they want.
5. The person you're in a relationship with plays mind games to portray themselves as a victim.

If you see any of these patterns at work in your relationships, ask yourself, "Does this person want me? Or do they want what I can do for them?"

Manipulation is an infection filled with deception, and it will not be long before the relationship becomes extremely unhealthy or ends in destruction.

If you're in a relationship, the other person should know your weaknesses, not to exploit them, but to cover them. If your weaknesses are being exploited, the soul tie is unhealthy. If this person is aware of your insecurities but refuses to protect them and instead compounds them, the soul tie is unhealthy. If this person talks you into giving up something important to you to make you more dependent upon them and then makes you feel bad for depending on them, the soul tie is unhealthy. These are examples of acts of manipulation that will lead to the other person controlling you.

"Intimidation" means "to make timid or fearful,"[6] and this is another form of control. When intimidation is present in a relationship, abuse is not far away. Intimidation happens by way of verbal or physical abuse or threats. Anytime you are afraid your mate is going to leave you or separate from you; you will accept threats, as well as verbal and psychological abuse.

When a clash between a dysfunctional couple occurs, it's common that one party will use manipulation and/or intimidation to get the other party to do what they want.

The following are five signs to help you recognize when intimidation is present in a relationship:

1. One member of a covenant relationship is afraid to make eye contact with the other person.
2. One person in the relationship doesn't speak up for what they want and caters to their mate's wants instead.
3. One person is reluctant to give constructive feedback, fearing the mate's hostile response.
4. One person suffocates or dilutes the greatness of their mate.
5. One person is irritated by the recognition and accolades of their mate, which makes that mate afraid to celebrate their own accomplishments.

Intimidation is an enemy to any relationship because it's counterproductive to the covenant relationship. The person who is intimidated (the victim) by the mate isn't free to express sincere and authentic love because fear is ever-present. 1 John 4:18 says, *"There is no fear in love; but perfect love casteth out fear because fear hath torment. He that feareth is not made perfect in love."* If intimidation is anywhere within a relationship, fear isn't far away.

The final element of control in unhealthy relationships is domination, which means "having a commanding influence on, exercise control over; to overlook from a superior elevation or command because of a superior position."[7]

When domination is present in a relationship, it's no longer a relationship but has instead become a dictatorship. One of Satan's major desires is to dominate every dimension of your life. If he sees you allowing another person whom you're in a relationship with to dominate you in some way, then he will try everything in his power to persuade that person to dominate you in all ways. Satan's goal is not only to make you miserable but also to make the dominator miserable.

If you feel powerless in your relationship, chances are good your mate is exercising dominance over you.

The following are seven signs of domination in a relationship:

1. Your mate makes you feel lesser than them.
2. You feel like you must walk on eggshells for fear of being abandoned.
3. Your mate gives you the evil eye, expecting you to respond in fear.
4. Your mate snaps at you in a group setting for having a different opinion from theirs.
5. You express feelings of hurt to your mate, but they shrug them off and demand, "Get over it!"
6. Your mate constantly corrects you in public in a hostile or disrespectful way.
7. Anytime something goes wrong, your mate blames you —even though the situation may not have anything to do with you.

It's one thing not to know about soul ties, but it's different to see the effects of ungodly and unhealthy soul ties and deny their existence. When the enemy's plots and schemes are revealed, but you stay in denial, that's consistent with rejecting God's Word. The second part of Hosea 4:6 speaks about rejecting knowledge: *"Because thou have rejected knowledge, I also will reject thee, that thou shalt be no priest to Me."* It sounds like God the Father is angered when He tries to enlighten us, but we reject His Knowledge.

One of the easiest ways to stay in bondage is to stay in denial. Let's return to Samson to see this at work in his life. Because Samson was in denial of his ungodly soul tie with Delilah, it led to his destruction. Once Samson was born into the world, his God-given purpose was to deliver God's people out of the bondage of their oppressor, the Philistines.

Because God had set apart Samson for this purpose, God gave specific instructions to Samson's parents so that their son would live a clean and powerful life. His parents were not to allow a razor to come upon his head, not to allow him to drink wine, not to allow him to eat unclean food, and not to allow him to take a wife from any of the heathen nations.

As soon as Samson came of age, he rebelled against the instructions of his parents and God, particularly by choosing a Philistine woman as his wife. Because God was determined to make all things work together for Samson's good, He allowed him to have the Philistine woman for the opportunity to destroy the Philistines.

After Samson married his first Philistine wife, they had a feast for seven days with 30 Philistine men attending. At the feast, Samson posed a riddle to the Philistines. They made a deal that if they could solve the riddle within seven days of the feast, Samson would give them 30 linen garments and 30 changes of clothes. But if they couldn't solve the riddle, they had to give Samson 30 linen garments and 30 changes of clothes.

For three days the men puzzled over the riddle but could not solve it. Without Samson's knowledge, on the seventh day, the Philistines went to Samson's wife and told her that if she didn't get Samson to explain his riddle to her and then give the answer to them, they would set fire to her and her father's house. Samson's wife manipulated him into giving her the meaning of the riddle, which she then passed on to the Philistine men.

The men came to Samson on the seventh day with the answer to the riddle. Samson got extremely angry and told them that they "solved" the riddle only because they had stolen it from his wife. The Spirit of the Lord came upon Samson, and he went down to another Philistine city, killed 30 men, stripped them, and gave their linen garments and changes of clothing to the men. Samson was so angry over his wife's betrayal that he went back to his father's house and separated from his wife (Judges 14).

Samson continued terrorizing the Philistines, but while doing so, he developed a bad habit: continually falling in love with Philistine women. Remember, these women were unclean, and he had been forbidden to marry them. Since Samson couldn't control his attractions, he found a Philistine harlot (i.e., prostitute) and had sexual relations with her.

Then he met Delilah, who he thought was the love of his life. *Delilah* means "head of hair."[8] That's exactly how she manipulated, intimidated, and dominated Samson. The Philistines knew they couldn't defeat Samson without knowing where his supernatural strength came from. When the Philistines saw how he loved Delilah, they knew she was their only hope of discovering Samson's strength. After Samson had developed a soul tie with Delilah, she made an agreement with the Philistine men to betray him for 700 pieces of silver.

Delilah said to Samson, "Please tell me where your great strength lies and with what you may be bound to afflict you?" Samson lied to her, though she didn't realize it, and she told the Philistines what Samson had said.

As he was asleep, she bound him up with strings and shouted, "The Philistines are upon you, Samson!" He jumped up, breaking the strings as a strand of yarn breaks when it touches fire. The ploy didn't work, but it showed Samson that Delilah was trying to betray him and kill him. Because he had a heavy ungodly soul tie, Samson remained in denial.

Delilah asked Samson three times about the source of his strength, and he lied three times. She tested him to see if he was telling her the truth by calling Samson out of his sleep, saying, "The Philistines are upon you!" He would jump up, looking for the Philistines, but they were never in sight. Instead of Samson recognizing she was trying to set him up to be killed and then walking away, he remained in denial. Then tragedy struck.

Delilah said to Samson, "How can you say I love you when your heart is not with me? You've lied to me three times and have not told me where your great strength lay."

Delilah kept pressing Samson—until his soul was vexed to death. Then finally, he told her the truth about his birth, his calling, and where his strength lay.

When Delilah felt he had told her everything in his heart, she sent for all the Philistine lords, saying, "Come up once more, for he told me everything in his heart."

So, the Philistines came and brought her the money. That night, Samson fell asleep with his head on Delilah's lap. She called for a man to shave off the seven locks on Samson's head.

Instantly, Samson's strength left, and Delilah screamed, "Samson, the Philistines are upon you!"

Samson jumped up and said, "I will go out as before and other times and shake myself free!"

Sadly, he didn't know that the Spirit of the Lord had left from him.

The Philistines grabbed Samson, gouged out his eyes, bound his hands and feet, and took him prisoner. This was the result of him remaining in denial about the ungodly soul tie with Delilah.

Anytime you have ignorance or when you're in denial about an ungodly soul tie, the enemy has you in the grip of deception. The enemy wants you tied to an ungodly soul tie so he can deceive you through your weak and desperate emotions. When you accept the deception, you become ineffective as a Christian.

If I could've sat down and interviewed Samson about the validity of ungodly soul ties, I believe Samson would've said this about his soul tie with Delilah: "I just did not know that ungodly soul ties were real."

CHAPTER 7

SECRET #2—THE ENEMY WANTS TO WOUND YOUR SOUL

WE MUST REMAIN aware that Satan is highly intelligent. He's a spiritual being who operates from the spirit world. Therefore, he has more knowledge about spiritual things than any human being who isn't connected to the Spirit of God. Remember, soul ties are first spiritual, before you see their effects in the physical.

The enemy isn't ignorant that God the Father is the Creator of soul ties. Satan knows who's the boss, and that anything God the Father creates is established forever because He is all-powerful. Therefore, the enemy doesn't try to stop God the Father from creating things, but he does try to infect and pervert what God the Father creates.

The enemy also knows that godly soul ties are unstoppable. When God the Father ordains, connects, and blesses a married couple, the enemy understands that if the couple remains in unity, follows the direction of God, and brings the best out of each other, then nothing he can do will destroy their union. The only way he can bring down the marriage is to infect their connection with so much offense that they will agree to divorce, thus wounding their souls.

When you examine your past friendships, partnerships, relationships, and family ties, you'll see that some of them were divine and God-ordained. How close were you two? Are you still close? If not, what happened to cause your friendship, relationship, or family tie to lose that closeness? Were you offended? Or did you offend that person? Whatever took place, something happened from the outside that caused offense, bitterness, strife, anger, or hurt to get inside the relationship. From there, you decided to cut ties with each other. I'm sure when you severed the friendship or relationship, it wounded someone's soul—or even both your souls.

As a pastor, I counsel, advise, repair, and reconcile a lot of relationships. They range from married couples to siblings, fathers and sons, mothers and daughters, boyfriends and girlfriends, and best friends. One day, I got a call from a great friend, asking me if I had time to help a friend of his, who was suffering from church hurt. I deal with that issue so much that I was reluctant. Then he told me that the guy had a background like mine. Instantly, my heart was pricked, so I made an exception.

An hour later, I was on the phone with my friend's friend, whose name was Matt. Matt was a 35-year-old former gang member and drug dealer who had been in prison for three years. He turned his life around and started living a Christlike lifestyle. Matt shared one of his struggles in the past. He was womanizing and having relationships with multiple women. Matt was a playboy until he had an encounter with Jesus in prison.

A few months after Matt got out of prison and started attending this church. The first Sunday he attended, the Holy Spirit was moving in powerful ways, and the pastor preached a dynamic word that made him feel like the sermon was speaking directly to him. On that Sunday, Matt joined the church, got connected to the men's ministry, and instantly became part of the fellowship.

A month later, Matt bought into the church mission, started serving on the parking lot ministry, and volunteered wherever the church needed help. Matt had an explosive personality, so the church loved him, and the pastor embraced him; he could see that Matt had a call on his life.

Matt said he was extremely faithful and available to the church. Then after two years, the church hired him. After a year of working at the church, Matt started dating a well-known lady in the church.. According to Matt, they dated for just a little over a year, but because they weren't compatible enough in certain areas, they mutually called it quits and went their separate ways.

A few months later, a rumor started spreading around the church that Matt had cheated the young lady out of $10K. Matt denied all the allegations, but the people in the church believed her. Matt said this young lady found out that he had taken another young lady in the church on a date, and this upset her, which was why she started the rumor.

It didn't take long for the people in the church to give Matt the cold shoulder. Matt said he went to the pastor to intervene, but the pastor refused to meet with Matt and his accuser. Weeks later, Matt said he came into a staff meeting a couple of minutes late, and the pastor embarrassed him by talking to him as if he were a child.

A few months later, the church fired Matt, which led to financial instability for a couple of months. Even after Matt got fired, he kept a strong connection to the church and the mission. Matt explained that he loved his church, the people, and his pastor. He found a new job, kept tithing, and he continued inviting people to church regardless of what happened in the past.

The final blow came when Matt said the pastor preached a sermon entitled "Preying on Your Pockets." It focused on advising women not to trust men who weren't as financially stable as them. Matt believed the pastor was referring to him, even though he never asked to hear Matt's side of the story.

Hurt, pain, and offense began to take root in Matt's heart. He wanted to stay connected to the church because the Word was feeding him, but deep down inside, he knew the church and pastor wouldn't accept him. Finally, Matt left the church. He didn't leave healed; he left hurt. Matt didn't leave better; he left bitter. He never got to converse with the pastor, and he never got the opportunity to clear his name. He cut ties with the church. His spirit was crushed, and his soul was shattered.

Here is the point: what God had connected and created between Matt and the church was a godly soul tie. As soon as persecution, lies, accusations, and offense got inside of Matt's heart, what was once godly turned ungodly. After being offended, every time Matt went to church, he couldn't receive the Word. He left empty, and he never felt the family touch he used to feel from the first time he visited.

At the end of our conversation, Matt said, "I am not ever going to another church! I'm not ever getting close to another pastor, and I don't want anything else to do with church folks!" What caused such a reaction? Anytime Satan sees a godly soul tie, his secret is to infect the cord (that ties people together) and wound the soul.

There are a few indications that will let you know when a person has a wounded soul. The first is unhealthy anger. Throughout my conversation with Matt, I could tell he was livid, infuriated, and irate. His anger had gotten so strong; it turned unhealthy during the conversation.

The Bible says, *"Be angry and sin not"* (Ephesians 4:26). Life happens, and our emotions can flare into anger, but you decide whether your anger will be healthy or unhealthy. Healthy anger is feeling the emotion yet keeping self-control and continuing to make healthy decisions. Unhealthy anger is feeling the emotion, yet losing self-control, thereby driving you to make unhealthy decisions.

In Matt's case, the healthy decision would've been to assess the situation and refuse to allow the lies from the young lady and the rejection from the pastor to cause him to develop hate for all church people or the church in general. Because one church group hurt him, doesn't give him the right to assume all church groups will hurt him.

Because of Matt's experience with one pastor, he developed a belief system that all pastors are the same. Instead of control-ling anger, he allowed unhealthy anger to control him. Unhealthy anger will control you when you're fearful and when you feel powerless in a situation or a soul tie.

The root of all unhealthy anger is a sense of powerlessness. When a person feels a lack of control in a situation, unhealthy anger can grow. As it continues to grow, it will turn into rage, bitterness, hatred, and unforgiveness. Anytime anger isn't responsibly managed, it will eventually wound your soul. It's

Satan's desire for you to live in a place of hurt without ever healing.

The second indicator of a wounded soul is nastiness. Anytime your soul is wounded, you feel like you must be nasty to people because you don't want anyone to get close to you. They might hurt you and reopen an old wound.

As I spoke with Matt over a series of conversations, trying to help him, he often got nasty with me. As I asked him questions and tried to lead him into healing, he assumed I was trying to get close to him. Therefore, he spouted nasty remarks.

Some people are "aggressive nasty," which means they are so hurt that when someone tries to be nice to them, their nastiness is immediate and aggressive. They want you to know that they're not concerned about having any new friends or associates.

Others are "nice nasty." They've mastered an outward smile, but spit sarcastic disrespect and verbal hate. They may smile while they're intimidating you or even be passive aggressive. They are unpleasant and spiteful towards people they don't know, and they do it all with poise, but the undertone is nasty.

The third indicator of a wounded soul is bitterness. Bitterness is a feeling of lasting anger and resentment caused particularly by perceived unfairness in suffering or by adverse circumstances.

Recall the story of Ruth and her mother-in-law Naomi. When Naomi's husband and two sons died, she told people, "Don't call me Naomi, but call me Mara, because the Lord has dealt bitterly with me." The name *Mara* means "bitter."[1] Because she felt that God had treated her unfairly and made her suffer the adverse circumstances of death, she had lasting anger and resentment. This name change from Naomi to Mara indicates a wounded soul.

Anytime I think about my conversation with Matt, I realize one of the traits of bitterness is that it drives us to be angry at everyone. It stems from bitterness from what the last person did to us. Bitterness loves company.

As I was trying to get Matt on the road to freedom by giving him wise counsel, he assumed I was trying to take up for the pastor. He started naming all the flaws the pastor had. Matt wanted me to see the pastor in the same light he saw the pastor so I would be angry with him because of how he had hurt Matt.

The Bible says, *"Lay aside bitter words, temper tantrums, revenge, profanity, and insults"* (Ephesians 4:31 [TPT]). Here, we see some of the traits that bitterness can produce. Matt was holding onto lasting anger; therefore, he had a temper tantrum during our conversation. He got upset because I wasn't angry at the pastor and didn't side with him about the situation.

Revenge is another fruit that comes from bitterness. If Matt would've had the opportunity to see the pastor on the day that I was talking to him, I believe he would've tried to get into a physical altercation with him. It was clear that Matt wanted revenge. If Matt didn't find a way to forgive the pastor, then he would wish nothing but the worst for the pastor.

You know bitterness is festering in your heart when you don't want the best for a person who has offended you. Not only did Matt want revenge, but he was so bitter he started using profanity in our conversation. When we had first started conversing, Matt was very respectful— until I touched those places of pain in his wounded soul.

Bitterness will cloud your perspective. Refusing to forgive is an indicator of a wounded soul. Matt was so hurt that he saw life through the lens of hurt and bitterness. Seeing life from a bitter perspective allows us to see only the worst in people and never consider seeing the best in them. Anytime the enemy sees that you've made it to that point, he will try to get you to the fourth and final sign of a wounded soul: unforgiveness. We will discuss forgiveness and unforgiveness in detail in Chapter 15.

Throughout this chapter, I've been using the term *wounded soul*. A person who has a wounded soul tends to carry the "voice of the victim," and see life from a broken perspective, and allows shame to shape their life.

The voice of the victim is a mouth that refuses to take responsibility for a mindset that has secretly accepted defeat. Because Matt felt defeated and powerless, in his heart he had secretly accepted the lie of defeat that the enemy was replaying in his mind. Because Matt had secretly accepted defeat, he was making excuses and living from a mindset of entitlement.

You may be wondering how one would not be defeated in this situation. One way to look at it is that in life, we don't win some and lose some; rather, we win some and learn something. In the instance of church hurt, it's not about winning and losing, it's about wisdom in learning.

Jesus said, *"In the world, ye shall have tribulation, but be of good cheer; I have overcome the world"* (John 16:33). In life things will happen that are beyond our control. Though we can't control everything that happens to us, we can control how we respond to it.

From Matt's point of view, he was lied about, wrongfully fired from his job, and treated inappropriately—all without having an opportunity to defend himself. To a degree, I believe that's true, but his focus shouldn't have been on what happened to him; rather, his focus should've been on not allowing anger, bitterness, nastiness, and unforgiveness to get inside him.

Throughout our conversation, he continued to place the blame on the young lady's lies and on the pastor for taking her side. I desperately tried to help Matt admit that it was his choice to get into the relationship with the young lady. Also, I tried to help him understand that it was his choice to break off the relationship and date another woman. Was he wrong? No, but his choices led to the young lady responding as she did—regardless of whether she was right or wrong. For Matt to start his healing process, he had to take ownership of and responsibility for the part he played, and the choices he made. No matter how it ended, he made his choices. It was difficult for Matt to see it that way. He didn't want to see how his choices played a key role in the outcome. If you can't see how your choices played a role in developing the soul tie that you're wrestling with you will remain tied. Ownership always leads to freedom.

Matt's conversation was one of continuing excuses and blaming. When I told Matt he wasn't the victim and how God was trying to teach him some wisdom in the situation, he turned on me. Because he felt entitled to an apology from the pastor for firing him and not listening to his side of the story, Matt refused to release the voice of the victim. This is one way I discovered that Matt had a wounded soul.

When people speak from the voice of the victim, they usually see life from a broken perspective. Everything is broken and is not fixable. Because their hearts are broken, they focus only on protecting themselves from disappointment in every circumstance and situation they encounter. Deep down in their hearts, they are living in shame, thinking everyone sees them as a broken person. Since they see themselves from a broken perspective, they believe everyone else sees them through the same broken and shattered lenses.

When both parties in a relationship sever the soul tie, both will wound their souls. A wounded soul can result from family rejection, family or friendship abandonment, family betrayal, family embarrassment, or family injustice. Whether it's your church family or natural family, the enemy desires to steal, kill and destroy the family ties because he knows God the Father created godly soul ties for families to stay in unity.

I don't write this chapter from the standpoint of a theory but godly wisdom and experience. By any means necessary, the enemy wants his infection to produce family dysfunction. For years I lived with a wounded soul because of ongoing family dysfunction. My mom and I were at odds and couldn't see eye-to-eye on many issues. As my relationship with God grew, I allowed His Spirit, men of God, forgiveness and ongoing growth to repair and restore my wounded soul.

David prayed that the Lord would restore his soul (Psalms 23). The evidence of a restored soul is keeping your God-given identity, carrying the peace of God, expressing the joy of the Lord, and living without offense. It's possible to live these godly elements when we want the life that God has planned for us, rather than to demand justice because of the injustice an offender did to us. The number one element you must embrace is destroying selfishness and self-centeredness. If you can release entitlement and the desire to satisfy your need for an apology, Godly peace will be your portion.

Growth in the Lord will cause you to bless the ones who cursed you and pray for the ones who hurt you.

CHAPTER 8

SECRET #3—UNGODLY SOUL TIES DESTROY MARRIAGES

BY NOW YOU know that the enemy hates anything God the Father creates. He hates the world; he hates the people in the world; he especially hates the children of God. The enemy knows that we, the children of God, have been instructed to live a godly lifestyle in an ungodly world. To make it hard on us, he tries to make us question the possibility of living a godly life in such an ungodly environment.

In the vast social-media age that we are living in, it's a daily battle against the three classes of the world's system. If children of God are to live up to the standards of Heaven, then we must defeat the daily temptations of lust of the flesh, lust of the eyes, and pride of life (1 John 2:16). These are the three areas that the enemy uses to tempt the children of God to live ungodly lives.

The lust of the flesh is the desire to fulfill the passion of the ungodly nature, which is animosity against the will of God. Even though you and I are children of God, and we have the Spirit of God living inside of us, we are not relieved of having to control ungodly appetites that try to arise in us.

103

Lust of the eyes is the desire to be pulled and persuaded to perform an ungodly action for pleasure, which comes from the things we see. Lust of the eyes makes us see and want what may appear good, but it doesn't mean that what we lust for is good for us.

Last, the pride of life is being obsessed with having a high status or title among certain groups in society to feel important. Usually, this desire is found in those suffering from low self-acceptance, low self-belief, low self-confidence, low self-esteem, low self-respect, low self-love, low self-value, and low self-worth.

The enemy knows the strength and power of agreement that can exist between a married couple; therefore, he's on a collision course, trying to destroy every God-ordained marriage he can. He does this through lust of the eyes, lust of the flesh, and pride of life, which creates the appetite to develop an ungodly soul tie within a God-ordained union.

It is helpful to pause and understand the purpose of marriage. Most people love the thought of marriage a lot more than they care to understand the purpose of marriage. The purpose of marriage is to become one, to build a life bigger than the two can do alone, and to bless God's people and the world around you. When two people come together in holy matrimony, they agree to become one with each other.

Another way of saying this is that the wife is consenting to this vow: "I want to become my husband." Likewise, the husband is consenting to this vow: "I want to become my wife." Every time I marry a couple, I start the wedding with a firm understanding, not just from the bride and groom, but also from the audience. My favorite line is "Ladies and gentlemen, right before your very eyes and mine, this husband and wife are making a mutual agreement to each other saying, "I want to become you."

Once again, this is the purpose of marriage, coming directly from the Throne of Heaven: *"Therefore, shall a man leave his father and mother and shall cleave unto his wife, and they shall become one flesh"* (Genesis 2:24 [KJV]).

THE FOUR SEASONS OF LOVE

The two becoming one takes place during the four seasons of love. In spring, the couple joins together, and everything in their lives is budding. They have butterflies, they laugh at each other's corny jokes, and neither one can do anything wrong in the other one's eyes. The happiness, joy, love, and excitement flowing from the couple is contagious to everyone close to them. In this season of the marriage, love and lust are flowing effortlessly.

Then the season of summer sets in. Not only is the sexual chemistry heating up but also the friendship, the conversation, the closeness, and the family feel. Neither party wants to be anywhere without the other, and the two can't wait to fulfill each other's every desire.

The season of fall in the marriage approaches. This is when the two start to shed who they are and embrace the different parts of each other: attitudes, habits, ways, thoughts, beliefs, desires, motives, and dreams. During the fall season, both people see what parts of themselves they will keep, and what parts they must release to function and flow within the union.

It's common for friction to become clear in the marriage during this season. Friction is not always a terrible thing; it's evidence that the marriage is about to bear fruit. Even though each spouse doesn't want to take on the other's attitude or habits, one will emerge as the stronger and reach down to pull up the weaker for the sake of flow. When one person doesn't want to become a specific part of the other, friction can occur. Sometimes, the fall season can last longer than the other three seasons because both parties are resisting the final season.

In the winter season of marriage, things start to die. Anytime a person's ways, attitudes, or preferences must die, it may cause an internal war between the two. Most couples want peace and camaraderie with each other, so this dying of self can be long and hard or short and sweet, depending on the couple's level of immaturity, stubbornness, and selfishness.

This is where sacrifice is either embraced or rejected. The only way a marriage can get out of winter is if both parties are willing to experience death of the self (i.e., sacrifice what they want for what their spouse wants). Therefore, I believe that true love will always make a sacrifice when no one else will.

The greatest encouragement of the winter season of love is that the couple knows spring is just around the corner. In marriage, these four seasons of love are always in rotation because God uses these four seasons so the two can become one flesh.

The second purpose of marriage is to build something bigger than the two can do alone. The phrase *"marriage is hard work,"* refers to the work of two people building something bigger than their individual selves in the midst of becoming one another.

Usually during the building process (because it's new, authentic, and original) things get a little complicated because no one has ever built your marriage. Yes, people have built marriages, but they haven't built your marriage. In the building phase, husband and wife must discover what works best for them. Just because certain things work for someone else's marriage doesn't necessarily mean it's going to work for every marriage.

From day one, my wife and I have had only one bank account. All our money goes into one account, and neither of us has any other separate accounts. In our six years of marriage, we've never had a financial problem, and we've always been financially stable and strong. On the other hand, I've counseled a lot of couples who won't consider combining their accounts. To be honest, I used to advise against a couple that has separate accounts—until I grew to understand that what works for us doesn't always work for others. Everyone's level of self-control and discipline is not the same, and this is also true of their finances.

Not only are you building a marriage, but a marriage is the building of a family. The Word of God says, *"So God created man in His own image, in the image of God, He created him; male and female, He created them, then God blessed them, and God said unto them, 'Be fruitful and multiply'"* (Genesis 1:27-28). This is where God instructs humankind to build a family.

Not only is marriage the tool God uses to build a family but also the tool God uses to build a business. In business, you serve people and build wealth. Likewise, marriage is the tool God uses for two people to build wealth. It takes teamwork, unity, wisdom, creativity and vision to build a successful business. When the two becomes one in those areas, married couples are unstoppable in business. Why? Because their oneness and agreement demands for Heaven's Spirit to rest upon them.

God uses marriage to build his church and advance his kingdom. When I met my wife and after our first conversation, she said that God gave her an open vision that we would build a church and take the gospel to the nations. Since we've been in ministry, God has used us to build people, repair marriages, and transform lives. The purpose of marriage is to build. Anytime a marriage doesn't build something, that marriage has an open door for the enemy to come in and attack it.

The Bible says, *"Where there is no vision, the people perish"* (Proverbs 29:18). Marriage is made up of two people with one vision. If the marriage doesn't have a vision, it won't be long before it perishes. Maybe the two people don't divorce, but both are lifeless and miserable. They are together on the outside but perishing on the inside. Vision will bring life back into the marriage. Gaining a vision of what God wants to build through their union, the couple's marriage will revive and bring purpose to it. Some marriages are unhealthy and dysfunctional because of a lack of vision; they don't have anything to build.

The third purpose of marriage is for the union to be a blessing. The word "bless" means "an empowerment to accelerate, increase, multiply, and succeed." This is why Solomon said, *"Whoso findeth a wife findeth a good thing and obtaineth favor of the Lord"* (Proverbs 18:22). When two people come together in holy matrimony, which has been approved by and given to Heaven, God the Father releases His Spirit upon them and places His Spirit into the marriage. His Spirit empowers them to increase, accelerate, multiply, and succeed. This union, partnership, and submission blesses not only the married couple, but others as well. When a marriage is divine (i.e., when it has been put together and approved by God), it will have a purpose, which will inspire, empower, and give hope to others.

Since the day my wife and I came together in marriage, we chose to do it God's way. We went against societal norms and followed the instructions of heaven. A week doesn't go by that someone doesn't tell us corporately or individually that our marriage gives them hope. Because society is pulling away from the biblical mandate of marriage, people are buying into the lie that "marriage isn't for everyone." My question to the people who are brave enough to make that statement to me is, "So fornication is for everyone? Because you do know that everyone you fornicate with, you're also creating an ungodly and unhealthy soul tie with them?" For 95% of couples who are not married but living as though they are, they are fornicating and creating multiple soul ties without ever being delivered from past soul ties.

I hope the people who admire our marriage tell themselves that it's possible to have a holy marriage in an unholy society. I hope our marriage inspires others to seek their lifelong mate. When a single person knows it's possible for peace and productivity to flow from a marriage, it pushes them to start looking for their own God-ordained marriage. The inspiration of being a power couple is contagious. God has empowered our marriage to empower others.

This is why the enemy hates marriage and godly soul ties; because when the partnership produces a purpose, it destroys dysfunction, unfruitfulness, and ungodliness. Anytime the enemy finds divinely inspired marriages, he looks for ways to destroy them by any means necessary. The most common ways are adultery and infidelity. What happens in the spirit realm when adultery and infidelity take place in marriage?

We've already established the fact that when two people come together in holy matrimony under the divine instructions of God, a godly soul tie has been formed. The Holy Spirit becomes a part of the threefold cord and He joins in the marriage with both parties. Some people undervalue His presence in marriage, but He's the most powerful part of the union. The bible says, *"Though one may be overpowered, two can defend themselves. A cord of three strands is not quickly broken"* (Ecclesiastes 4:12 [NIV]).

The cord of three strands is God, the groom, and the bride. The braiding of these three strands together symbolizes the joining of the couple and God in marriage. When two people keep Jesus at the center of the marriage and allow the Holy Spirit to be the Supreme Governor, the love of God will continue to grow in the marriage and bind the couple together.

The enemy knows that once a marriage is committed to the authority of heaven, that marriage will bring destruction to his kingdom. Therefore, he looks for any opportunity to tempt either the husband or the wife (or both) with the lust of the flesh, the lust of the eyes, or the pride of life. If the temptation is accepted, the enemy ties an ungodly cord from an outside person to the godly cord of either the husband or wife.

If this takes place, then an ungodly cord has been bound to a godly cord. At that point, the marriage doesn't have the godly cord of the Holy Spirit that it was once bound with because the Holy Spirit has left. Whoever allowed the ungodly cord to come in wasn't being obedient to the Governor's (i.e., the Holy Spirit's) promptings, nudging, or convictions, and thus dismissed the godly cord. The Holy Spirit left because He didn't agree to a four-fold cord, an ungodly cord, or the rejection of His Voice. Whoever the victim is may have not been initially aware of what happened, but eventually they will discover that the Holy Spirit is not reigning over the marriage.

This reminds me of Minister Mike, a former colleague I met in 2012 after I preached at a church in Atlanta, Georgia. For a brief period, I became great friends with Minister Mike. When he and I met, Minister Mike was highly inspired by the message I gave and asked if I would mentor him in the Word of God. Around that time, Minister Mike was 32 years old and about to be elevated to Assistant Pastor at his church.

Minister Mike had been happily married for six years. He and his wife had two sons, had just bought their first home, and were doing very well financially in corporate America. Minister Mike had a passion to learn the Word of God, and a deep desire to become a full-time pastor.

For two years, we talked once a week, and at every opportunity, he came to hear me preach or speak whenever I was in Georgia. In 2015, I moved to Houston, and Minister Mike had been promoted to a full-time pastor.

Now, Pastor Mike had been the Senior Pastor at his church for about 18 months. Unexpectedly, he called me and told me to pray for him. Initially, I assumed pastoring and working a full-time job were starting to weigh heavily on him. Therefore, I encouraged him to endure the season of stagnation.

What hit me like a ton of bricks was when Pastor Mike said, "James, I don't need you to pray about the frustrations of a small church because what I didn't tell you is that in the last 18 months, the church has grown from about 60 people to 400 people every Sunday morning. What I need you to pray about is that I think I'm falling in love with another woman."

As soon as I heard what he said, it felt like a golf ball had gotten stuck in the back of my throat. I took a deep breath and said, "What?"

Pastor Mike responded, "Bro, I told you because I didn't think you would judge me. James, please, I need you to be my friend and not my mentor or my judge."

I paused for a second to gather my thoughts. "Mike, open rebuke is better than secret love. Bro, I wouldn't be your friend if I didn't tell you that you're deceived. No way you should be comfortable telling anybody to pray for you because you think you're in love with another woman. Prayer will not solve the problem, only repentance will. I'm not judging you, but I am inspecting your fruit and giving you truth."

Pastor Mike hung up on me. About six months later, I got word that Pastor Mike was stepping down from pastoring the church after a two-year stint. He had been caught and admitted to having an adulterous affair with another woman, but the main reason the church made him step down was that he had told the church board that he was leaving his wife and marrying his lover.

Every time I'm reminded of this, it shows me just how intentional the enemy is about destroying a godly marriage. Lust of the flesh, lust of the eyes, and pride of life made Minister Mike give the enemy an opportunity to destroy a godly marriage and a godly family by way of an ungodly soul tie. To this day, I am clueless how Pastor Mike met his lover—who, to my knowledge, is still his current wife—but how it happened doesn't matter; Pastor Mike allowed himself to be connected to an ungodly soul tie that was outside his godly marriage. As soon as Pastor Mike developed an ungodly soul tie and brought it into his marriage, the Holy Spirit left the marriage. The Holy Spirit never agreed to a four-fold cord; He agreed to a threefold cord. As soon as the Holy Spirit left the marriage, Pastor Mike was no longer being led by the Holy Spirit but by lust of the flesh, lust of the eyes, and pride of life.

The enemy wasn't only trying to destroy the marriage; he also succeeded in wounding Pastor Mike's children. The divorce—which was driven by an ungodly soul tie—hurt his two sons.

The enemy will use anything or anyone to destroy a godly union and make it ungodly—especially lust of the flesh, adultery, and an ungodly soul tie.

Husbands and wives, be careful because the enemy would love to destroy your marriage by way of an ungodly soul tie.

CHAPTER 9

SECRET # 4—THE ENEMY WANTS YOU TO CHO OSE A PERSON BEFORE YOU DISCOVER YOUR PURPOSE

FOR THE LAST SIX YEARS, I've had the privilege of pastoring Transforming Faith Christian Center in Houston, Texas. From day one, it's been one of the most fulfilling assignments of my life. We have a fivefold message we preach and teach. Our mission is to reach the lost, train the ones who've been reached, and release the trained to go out and advance heaven's kingdom agenda.

Anytime you come through the doors or listen to us by way of social media, you'll always receive a message on either transformation, vision, encouragement, identity, or faith. God has chosen us to take people from–to. We are taking people from brokenness to wholeness; from a defeated mindset to a victorious mindset. We are taking people from hurting to healing; from chaos to peace; from a poverty mindset to a prosperous mindset. We are taking people from trauma to triumph, from religion to relationship, from immaturity to maturity, from no vision to full vision, and from being indifferent to having a passionate life.

For four and a half years, I taught these messages and directed them toward finding God's purpose for our lives, living fearlessly, and having an overall desire to change one's life for the better. God's hand is certainly on our church, but in the last year and a half, God has been breathing the winds of acceleration upon us.

What has accelerated the momentum of our church is in the area of relationships and marriage. It took four and a half years for this to begin because I felt like I was struggling between teaching people what they need versus what they want to hear.

I felt like all people wanted to hear were sermons on relationships. They would take the principles back into their relationships, and use the information on the person they're with, hoping to change them. Most people refuse to examine themselves first before trying to point out what's wrong with their mate. I've always lived by this: No one needs to get into a relationship until first they have a secure relationship with themselves. Therefore, I neglected the relationship sermons until my wife opened my eyes to see how many people were hurting personally, financially, spiritually, and emotionally simply because of a broken heart that came from a failed relationship.

As soon as the people started consistently hearing our relationship wisdom, the momentum exploded. I created a TikTok page that forced me to keep posting relationship content. I built a following of 200K+ people in nine months.

My counseling sessions have increased dramatically, my mentoring sessions are at an all-time high, and my inbox messages are overflowing from people who want relationship advice. Anytime I counsel or advise a single person who wants to know why it is so hard to make the right choice in dating, relationships, and marriage, I consistently say, "Never choose a person who doesn't have a great feel for their purpose and never choose a person if you don't have a great feel for your purpose." If you choose the person before you discover your purpose and then later discover your purpose, the person may not want to go where your purpose is taking you. They may not be equipped with the proper tools to help you build your purpose. They may not like the person that your purpose is turning you into.

The fourth secret of the ungodly soul tie is that the enemy wants you to create a soul tie before you discover or start pursuing your God-given purpose. If the enemy can get you to think fleshly, he will press you into connecting with a person who will deter you from your destiny.

In August 2011, I walked out of prison with a new mind, a new perspective, a new mission, and a new purpose. I was excited to begin creating my new life. Months before being released, I rolled out the vision and the plan I had for my future. To my surprise, everything I planned went in the opposite direction of what I saw. I sat in prison for six years writing my life story of transformation. I planned to get out, get my book published, join a church, then go around the world telling my story and selling the book.

Sadly, when I got home, I discovered that everything I thought I had was gone. Plus, when I went to the church that I felt God had told me to go to, I was rejected. I experienced a little church hurt, and for a while, I couldn't connect to the right church home, but what I thought was a disaster turned out to be God's divine direction.

I had a great friend who played cornerback for the Houston Texans, a NFL team. When they entered training camp in July, every morning I would be on a conference call with him and the defensive backs, which was 10 people in total. I would motivate them to make the best of their opportunity to play professional football. Four weeks later, my friend flew me to Houston to attend their preseason game.

After the game, he and his crew of defensive backs introduced me to the General Manager and the Team Chaplain. They asked that I give a motivational message to the entire team. Two months later, the request was granted. A month later, I found myself in Jacksonville, Florida, giving a motivational message to the Houston Texans the night before they played the Jacksonville Jaguars.

That was not only a huge accomplishment for a man who had been out of prison for fewer than six months, but also a life-changing opportunity. After I gave the message to the team, the local newspaper from my hometown got wind of my story, checked the facts, and wrote my story of redemption on the front page of the newspaper. Instantly, I started receiving invitations for motivational speaking at middle schools, high schools, universities, nonprofit organizations, and churches all over the nation.

When the local church rejected me, the motivational speaking world accepted me. For the next year and a half, I traveled from city to city, state to state, and stage to stage telling my story. Though I didn't publish my book, God was allowing me to build an audience and credibility with influential people. I ended up being a keynote speaker at the Steve Harvey Boys Mentoring weekend in Dallas, Texas, for four years in a row.

I was focused, growing, and accelerating at a rapid pace. After one speaking engagement, I met a guy who was part-owner of a pharmaceutical company. He told me that the Spirit of God impressed him to fund my ministry. Since I was doing motivational speaking and didn't think I would ever be a pastor, I declined his offer. However, since I had built a connection with him, a few months later, he hired me as one of his pharmaceutical sales reps, while I continued my motivational-speaking career.

At that point, I felt like it was time to get into a relationship. I made two major mistakes: (1) I didn't consult with God, and (2) I was being led by fleshly thinking. Fleshly thinking is birthed from self-centered thinking. These are the thoughts that replay in our minds and sound like this: *"This is what I want; this is who I'm going to get, and this is who I'm going to be with."* It's a mistake to repeat and entertain these thoughts but never consider God's intentions to create a godly union. Therefore, we pursue what we want, when we want it, and how we want it.

I wasn't on social media just to stay current on the latest news, absorb godly content, and feed my good relationships, but I was also there to pursue who and what I wanted. I was a completely new person, empowered with a new purpose; therefore, it would've been wise to pursue a person who was on the same path as I was or had the same purpose I was pursuing, but I started dating a person who had the appetites and attractions of my past life, rather than the passion to join me on the pathway to purpose.

I was a man who had been in prison for six years and had to control my sexual appetite. Therefore, when I started dating this young lady, I never considered that not only would I have to continue controlling my sexual appetites and desires, but that I would also have to continue crucifying the old man ("Butch") whom I had buried.

Many people might say that since I'm a human being and had been in prison, having sex with a woman was not an issue. But please know that these are fleshly thoughts that can push us into rebelling against the Word of God. They are self-centered thoughts that train us to put what we want first, without even considering what God wants for us. From the depths of my heart, I was truly trying to live my life for Christ, but when I started embracing fleshly thinking, no longer was I willing to continue making godly sacrifices.

I didn't want people in my hometown to think that I hadn't changed, so I wouldn't take the young lady out on any local dates. Instead, we drove to Huntsville or Decatur, Alabama (an hour away), for our dates. At that time, I was still living at my grandmother's house. The young lady had three kids, so I couldn't go to her house until the kids went to sleep. Also, I had to make sure that my grandmother was asleep before I snuck out the door and went over to my girlfriend's house. I didn't want my grandmother to think I was doing anything that would lead me back into my past lifestyle. But more than this, sin brings shame. Therefore, I went to her house every night at about 11:30 and stay until about 2:30 in the morning.

As soon as the sex and emotional attachment got stronger, I stayed longer. 2:30 AM turned into 3:30 AM, and then into 4:30 AM, and then 5:30 AM. One morning, I snuck out the door after the kids' alarm clock went off.

A couple of hours later, I got a call from the pastor whose church I had been attending. "The word on the street is that someone saw you coming out of Barbara's house earlier this morning, and they told me that they watched you walk around the corner to the nursing home, where your car was parked. Please don't tell me that you're fornicating with Barbara, while you're out here doing ministry, too."

I was shocked! I couldn't believe someone had seen me come out of her house and go to my car. Instead of saying it wasn't me or that I didn't know what he was talking about, I said, "Yeah, Pastor, but what people don't know is that we got married about a week ago."

"What! James, are you serious? If you're married, then why are you parking the car around the corner at the nursing home?"

"Because she's not ready to tell her kids, and I'm not ready to tell anyone either. You're the first person who knows, so please keep it to yourself and don't tell anyone until we announce it."

He burst out laughing. "Well, congratulations, Minister Edwards! I pray that the two of you have a successful marriage."

Without Barbara's knowledge, she was suddenly married, and her last name was Edwards!

Five minutes later, I called Barbara and asked if we could have a serious face-to-face conversation. Of course, she agreed, so I drove to her house. As the conversation began, I expressed how God had convicted me about our sexual relationship. To my surprise, she said that God had been convicting her also, but she didn't know how to tell me.

That's when I told her, "I think we should get married."

She was shocked. Seconds later, she took a deep breath. "You really want to marry me?"

"I think we should do it because I can't keep on fornicating with you. And it's going to be hard to stop."

"Of course, I'll marry you! Let's set a date," Barbara said.

"Why we gotta wait? I think we can make this happen today," I said.

"How?"

"We can ride down to Franklin County and get the judge to marry us now."

Anxiety clouded her face. "Are you serious?"

"Absolutely."

Minutes later, Barbara and I were on the road, headed a couple of counties away to get married. After our courthouse marriage, we came back home. I needed to go to Huntsville, Alabama, to secure a speaking engagement. On the road to Huntsville, I received a call from the university's admin, telling me that I didn't need to come because they had canceled the event. I turned around, went back to Florence, and met with a friend to work on a new video.

I didn't go back to Barbara's house until about 11:30 that night. In my mind, we would discuss our plan to tell her kids that they had a stepfather, as well as figure out the best way to tell our families we had just gotten married. To my surprise, when I came in the door and walked into the bedroom, she wasn't there. I searched for her. Minutes later, I found her on the floor, curled up in her closet, sulking and crying.

I was shocked and concerned because I didn't know what was wrong. "Barbara! What's going on?"

She was shaking. "Y-you married me t-today but w-wouldn't even spend the day with me! You don't love me."

I was at a loss for words. As far as I was concerned, we hadn't talked about her introducing me to her kids, so how was I to know that I was supposed to spend the day with her? I stood in shock and tried to figure out why she had slipped into a deep depression in just a couple of hours since I had last seen her. My only thought was, *"What in the world have I gotten myself into?"*

Seconds later, a still, small voice entered my thoughts. *"Son, you can't cover up a mess; you have to repent from a mess. What you're trying to cover up secretly, I'm going to expose openly."* I knew it was the voice of God, but I didn't fully pay attention to it.

For the next 30 days, my life was a living hell. I was a pharmaceutical sales rep, and she was a cosmetologist. Therefore, I went to work early in the morning, and sometimes she stayed up working until 2 AM. I had trained myself to get up at 5:30 every morning for personal development and Bible-study time. Barbara hated that when she came home from work, I was asleep and refused to wake up and talk to her.

The kids' father saw me with her at their son's game and tried to embarrass me publicly. Before I knew it, people were between us, breaking up a potential fight. After that incident, I came to myself and realized that I was still on federal probation. If I went to jail, I would be sent back into federal prison on a probation violation.

I am not an argumentative type of person, but every single day in the marriage I was having to argue, fuss, and fight verbally to be respected and heard. It seemed as if the only time Barbara and I got along was when we were having sex or if I was doing exactly what she asked me to do and how she wanted me to do it.

Being a stepdad to the kids took a toll on me. Their dad had told them that they didn't have to respect me. About four months into trying to make the wrong marriage right, Barbara asked me to take her sons to a high school football game. I told her that if they wanted to go to a game, they would have to go to the game I was going to. The kids got upset, I refused to take them to the game they wanted to go to, and I went to "my" game. After the game, I went to her salon to check on her and the kids. She exploded on me in front of about six of her clients. She ran up to me and screamed, "You stupid [bleep, bleep]! I'm sick and tired of you!"

My anger flared. I felt disrespected. "What!? Who are you calling stupid?"

"You! You ain't nothing but a punk [expletive]!" She was nose to nose with me and pointing her finger in my face.

I was tempted to slap her finger away from my face, but I saw the federal penitentiary in my mind's eye.

Then suddenly, I heard that still, small voice say, *"Leave. Don't let her trick you out of your future."*

As I was hearing that still small voice speak to me, she was still in my face pointing and provoking me. "What are you going to do now?" She added a few foul words to press her point.

I turned and walked away. "I'll be whatever you want me to be, but the one thing I won't be is a prisoner back in the penitentiary!" I shut the door after leaving, got into the car, and went to her house to pack up everything I owned. I left for good.

The marriage didn't last six months. The lust of the flesh, the lust of the eyes, and the pride of life tricked me into choosing a person who wasn't conducive to the purpose of God that was resting on my life. What do you do when you choose someone you think is best for you, then later you learn that God doesn't agree with your choice?

After we separated, I was forced to look at the situation through the eyes of truth rather than through the eyes of lust and sex. I noticed that I had created and married an ungodly soul tie.

I realized that every time I had a speaking engagement out of town, and Barbara couldn't attend, she would try to stop me from going by starting a fight with me. I recognized that she didn't value personal development, and if she thought I was reading or studying too much, then she viewed me as "lazy" and "slacking on family responsibilities." I saw clearly where my life was going, and she wasn't interested in becoming the person whom she had to be to get us there. She couldn't help me execute my assignment because she wasn't equipped with the necessary tools.

Please don't interpret this to mean that she was a terrible person. All I mean is that she wasn't the person who had the characteristics or the ability to help me build my purpose—my helpmate. I have since discovered, joy, peace, chemistry, part-nership, and happiness flow from God's purpose for marriage. When two people are united from heaven's instructions, building purpose is a part of the union. Good sex and the absence of purpose in a relationship or a marriage is a recipe for destruction.

As I was counting the cost of reconnecting and starting over again, I had more cons than pros. I felt as though something internally was pulling me to stay tied to someone who was destroying the potential of my destiny. As soon as I stopped thinking fleshly, I allowed the Spirit of God to direct me.

Lust and ungodly soul ties will force us to choose the person before discovering and pursuing our purpose. Instead, it is wise to discover our purpose, and then God will bring the person to us, who will come alongside us, as we move forward in our God-given purpose.

CHAPTER 10

SECRET #5—SOUL TIES ARE TOOLS FOR SPIRITUAL WARFARE

As I THINK BACK to every ungodly and unhealthy soul tie I was knitted and bonded to in the past, it's clear that these soul ties were the enemy's tools in spiritual warfare against me. Spiritual warfare is the struggle, the war, and the fight against unhealthy and ungodly soul ties. Biblically, spiritual warfare is referred to in Ephesians 6:10-18 and 2 Corinthians 10:3-6.

Engaging in spiritual warfare is not a matter of "if" but "when." On the day you accepted Jesus Christ as your personal Lord and Savior, you committed treason against the kingdom of darkness. You renounced your allegiance to darkness and announced your allegiance to the Kingdom of Light. Therefore, all of hell hates you.

You can see this clearly in Colossians 1:13: *"He has delivered us from the power of darkness and conveyed us into the Kingdom of the Son of His Love* [Jesus Christ]*"* (NKJV). This means that your decision to switch spiritual kingdoms to Jesus' created a life-long enemy of Satan. Satan views Jesus as his enemy; therefore, if you're part of Jesus' Kingdom, then Satan hates you. Whether you're a child of God or not, every day of your life, the enemy of your soul will try to oppress, suppress, or depress you by way of spiritual warfare.

For the child of God, Satan's agenda is to rob you of your freedom in Christ. The enemy can use ungodly and unhealthy soul ties to pull even a mature believer, who has a strong relationship with God and the Holy Spirit, away from the will of God.

If you've willingly made allegiance with an ungodly soul tie, you're in rebellion against God's desires for your life. Usually, most people know when they're connected to someone who's not going in the same direction as they are. As we've discussed earlier, the people they are connected to are not interested in growing into the next version of who God wants them to be in Christ. If you are connected to someone who doesn't want to grow, they will hinder your growth.

Even though you know the person isn't good for you, that doesn't mean you are willing to separate from them because you still want something from them. Often, people who are knowingly in an ungodly soul tie pray for God to change the person because they want that person to be who God wants for them, but as is so often the case, that person is not willing to make the changes or sacrifices necessary for the relationship to move from an ungodly connection to a godly connection. When friction in the relationship intensifies, spiritual warfare has begun. It starts as two people, each fighting for dominance or control over the other.

However, an unhealthy soul tie could have started healthy. Maybe you feel like God did send that person into your life, but it's not God's fault that the person chose to deviate from the principles of growth to become unhealthy to you. Please, never forget this principle. Write it in your journal or on a post-it note and review it often. "IT'S NOT GOD'S FAULT THAT THE PERSON CHOSE TO DEVIATE FROM THE PRINCIPLES OF GROWTH TO BECOME UNHEALTHY FOR YOU."

Sometimes we forget that the greatest gift God gave to us is the gift of choice. Likewise, the most dangerous gift God gave to us is the gift of choice. Therefore, if a person starts to be healthy for you but then makes unhealthy choices and thus becomes unhealthy for you, it's not God's fault. That person exercised free will to make those choices.

Consequently, this is how the enemy can use people as a tool for spiritual warfare. He doesn't want you to know that ungodly and unhealthy soul ties are his tools in spiritual warfare against you.

Spiritual warfare happens on the battlefield of the mind:

> "For although we live in the natural realm, we
> don't wage a military campaign employing
> human weapons, using manipulation to
> achieve our aims. Instead, our spiritual
> weapons are energized with divine power to
> effectively dismantle the defenses behind
> which people hide. We can demolish every
> deceptive fantasy that opposes God and break
> through every arrogant attitude that is raised
> up in defiance of the true knowledge of God.
> We capture, like prisoners of war, every
> thought and insist that it bows in obedience to
> the Anointed One. Since we are armed with
> such a dynamic weaponry, we stand ready to

punish any trace of rebellion as soon as you
choose disobedience."

— 2 CORINTHIANS 10:3-6 (TPT)

2 Corinthians 10:5 says, *"We can demolish every deceptive fantasy,"* which is an internal picture or thought of a lie that masquerades as the truth. Where is this thought or picture found? In the mind. It goes on to say that we break every arrogant attitude, which is a mindset that insults others because they believe they are better, smarter, or more important than other people. Where does this arrogant attitude begin? In the mind.

The end of 2 Corinthians 10:5 says, "We capture, like prisoners of war, every thought and insist that it bow in obedience to the anointed one." We capture every thought by being aware of the thoughts we think—in the mind. If the enemy can use an ungodly or unhealthy soul tie to oppress, suppress, or depress you, he must first get some control of your mind.

Therefore, oppression and suppression of the ungodly or unhealthy soul tie results in defeated thinking, depression, discouragement, despair, shame, pride, rebellion, arrogant thinking, deceptive fantasies, lack, poverty, debt, embarrassment, lack of purpose, illegitimate identity, unforgiveness, hate, religion, racism, superiority, racism, betrayal, rejection, abandonment, unworthiness, fear, loneliness, low self-esteem, insecurities, low self-value, low self-respect, unhealthy competition, low self-belief, guilt, low self-confidence, self-hate, double-mindedness, envy, jealousy, complacency, lack of faith, and unhealthy competition. That's quite a list of the effects of spiritual warfare when you're connected to ungodly or unhealthy soul ties.

Let me give you more information, so you can determine if you're in the midst of spiritual warfare with an unhealthy or ungodly soul tie.

You may feel worn down mentally, emotionally, and spiritually. This results from disagreements, bickering, arguing, verbal abuse, and/or feeling like you just can't do enough to satisfy your mate. This wears you down, and then the enemy wants to hear you say, *"I'm tired,"* because you don't have any fight left in you. When you say this but lack the desire to sever the soul tie, you're subconsciously giving the enemy permission to oppress, suppress, or depress you. *"I'm tired"* means that you don't believe the two of you can work together for the common good of the union. *"I'm tired"* means that you are out of patience to continue trying to change things.

If you are tired of the warfare but don't try to sever the soul tie, then eventually you will quit resisting the desires of the other person and accept the oppression. I can never forget the time when I was in prison, and my ex-girlfriend was pressing me about paying off the truck and signing it over to her. Deep down, I knew she wasn't going to remain loyal to me. I knew she would get the truck, and then stop accepting my phone calls. I knew it was time for me to let her go, but I was afraid because I was worried about what the people were going to say about me back home.

But she kept pressing me. Every time we talked, she hounded me. Eventually, I was worn out from her pressuring me about the truck and the fear of her leaving me. I gave in.

In spiritual warfare, if the enemy can wear you down, you'll end up tolerating disrespect, betrayal, disloyalty, and rejection. If this goes on long enough, you'll end up entertaining dysfunction.

Let me offer you a few signs that show when you're worn out:

1. **You get to the point where you dread having to interact with this person.** Maybe you're married; maybe you're living with your mate; maybe you are best friends or coworkers, or maybe you are family and have been close all your life. If you dread having any interactions with them, then they are wearing you down, and it won't be long before they wear you out. Somehow, someway, you have accepted their opposing behavior, habits, or ways without demanding that they change. What's inside them and attached to them has found a way to get inside you and attach itself to you. You don't want to tolerate their effects or opposing elements anymore, but instead of putting your foot down and confronting what you don't like, you continue to allow it—even while dreading it. The principle you did not consider is that whatever you tolerate will dominate you. You tolerated their negative conversation, selfishness, bad attitude, and laziness; therefore, all that has become a part of your life, and you don't like it. Instead of fighting against it openly, all you do is dread them internally. What's sad is that when you reach your breaking point, you're going to explode. Depending on your level of self-control, this explosion could turn into destruction. The goal of the enemy is to use others to wear you down, so you lose self-control.

2. **You feel like you always need to vent to others about the problems in your marriage or relationship.** Needing to vent to others instead of to your spouse or mate is because you feel they do not listen to or respect you. If this is the case, then it's typically because you're

not in a marriage or a relationship; rather, you're in a dictatorship. The other person has the control, and it's wearing you out. This is the enemy's strategy in warfare. He pressures you into accepting his suggestions. Next, it will produce oppression and suppression to wear you out. Most of the time, when you vent to others about your marriage or relationship problems, you tend to talk to people who are in the same circumstance or situation you are in. If they, too, are in a dictatorship and not a relationship, then they can't help you. All they can do is listen. You'll form friendships from the foundation of pain. If growth is your goal, then never discuss your problems with people who lack wisdom, because they can't empower you. The best they can do is enable you to stay the same. Instead, when you're in spiritual warfare, you need information and strategies that you can apply to your situation.

3. **You feel exhausted, sad, or anxious after interacting with them.** They make excessive withdrawals from you without depositing anything into you. One way to defeat your enemies is to strip them of the resources they need to fight against you. Likewise, in spiritual warfare, the enemy works to strip you of your confidence, joy, peace, and internal strength. If you're not confident, then you're insecure and suspicious. If you lack joy and are sad, then you'll eventually adopt a pessimistic mentality. If you don't have peace in the marriage or relationship, then you are living with chaos and confusion, thereby leaving you powerless.

4. **Finally, if you're not internally strong, then you'll be internally weak, and then you'll take on a victim mentality.** If the enemy can wear you out, then you're

no longer a threat to him, and you can't bring the best out of your mate.

I spent a lot of time exposing the enemy's tactic of wearing you out because it's effective and a priority of his agenda in spiritual warfare.

After you've been worn down and worn out by your mate, the next loss you're vulnerable to is losing the fire you once had for God. Anytime you lose your fire for the things of God, you're in the midst of spiritual warfare.

As a pastor, I've witnessed many single people who are on fire for the Lord come to the church. They worship, serve, and lead with an absolutely intoxicating fervor, but I've learned not to get too excited because if they start dating a person who is not on fire, then that person has the potential to suffocate their zeal.

The Bible says, *"Can two walk together—except they be agreed?"* (Amos 3:3); *"Bad company corrupts good character"* (1 Corinthians 15:33 [NLT]), and *"Be ye not unequally yoked together with unbelievers, for what fellowship hath righteousness with unrighteousness, and what communion hath light with darkness?"* (2 Corinthians 6:14). If the enemy can get you tied to a nonbeliever, then it won't be long before your fire sputters and dies. When that happens, you've lost a critical tool to untangle the soul tie.

If you are in a relationship with someone who is not on fire for God, then pay attention to their subtle attempts to isolate you from your church family. Don't be surprised if they ask, "Do you have to go to church every Sunday? Why do you have to go to Bible study every Wednesday night? Do you attend every small group meeting during the week? Don't you get tired of going to church? What do you get out of going to church? Don't they have someone else who can serve in your spot this Sunday?"

These questions show that as it pertains to the area of spirituality, they are not on the same page as you. It becomes dangerous when they make plans for you on the days you attend church functions, or when you're supposed to honor your commitment to serve. The enemy knows you want to be with your newfound friend or mate; therefore, he will push them to pressure you to spend time with them and minimize your time to connect with God. If you allow it, then the enemy will use this person to pull you away from your relationship with God and isolate you in a whole new world. This strategy from hell is being applied to your feelings and desires to annihilate you in spiritual warfare.

If you're with someone who's not driving you into a deeper relationship with God but pulling you away from God, you're in a dangerous situation. You cannot ignore what Jesus said in John 15:4: *"So, you must remain in the life union with Me, but I remain in life union with You, or as a branch separate from the vine will not bear fruit, so your life will be fruitless unless you live your life intimately joined to Mine"* (TPT).

Staying in union with Jesus is necessary. Anytime you develop a soul tie with someone who's not of the same spiritual mind as you, it won't be long before you are forced to choose between this person or God's purpose for you. You'll either allow your relationship with God to pull you away from this person or this person to pull you away from your relationship with God.

Therefore, it's wise to allow a mentor or spiritual guide to advise you before creating an unhealthy or ungodly soul tie. Sometimes, when we consistently make the wrong choices in a mate, it's wise to allow someone the space to "get into your business." When you are choosing a mate, you don't typically want people in your business. However, the same person you don't want in your business might be the one you need to call for advice after the heartbreak. What if you would've introduced your new friend to your mentor or spiritual advisor before you got emotionally attached? Maybe they could've pointed out the red flags that your hidden desires wouldn't let you see.

The enemy wants to put out your fire, so you'll quit on God. Therefore, the final element of spiritual warfare from an ungodly and unhealthy soul tie is when you contemplate giving up on God. When people arrive at this point, many entertain the thought that the situation is God's fault. They think, *"God, I can't believe you allowed them to do me like this,"* or, *"I fasted for this person, and now they betrayed me like this!"* They insinuate that God ordained it or didn't come to their rescue. They get upset with God, rather than themselves, so they can feel better about walking away from God.

The truth is, one of the scariest things about getting into a marriage or relationship, is that you must have faith that the person is honest and will do what they said they'd do and be who they said they'd be. This goes for you, too. The person whom you choose to marry or enter a relationship with must trust you in this same way. If either of you doesn't fulfill your promises, then it's not God's fault. What do you expect when you connect with a person who isn't being led, taught, consulted, or directed by the Word of God?

The enemy will send someone to attach to you who will steal your peace, kill your vision, and destroy your destiny. His assignment is not just to fight you but also to destroy you. That's why it's called spiritual warfare. If you get attached to an ungodly soul tie, no matter what it looks like or what it feels like, you're in the midst of spiritual warfare. Be wise as a serpent and harmless as a dove.

Now that you're armed with the knowledge of the strategies that Satan uses against you, you can avoid the spiritual warfare and damaging results of unhealthy and ungodly ties. Grab hold of wisdom to connect only to godly soul ties and live in victory!

CHAPTER 11

SECRET # 6—THE SOUL TIE WANTS TO STEAL YOUR IDENTITY

WHEN TWO PEOPLE in an ungodly or unhealthy soul tie desire to be free from each other but can't make the break, a mystery is at work. The question most people ask is, "How can I join myself with a person, then physically get released from the person but still be knitted or feel bonded to the person?" You opened yourself to the person physically by way of sex, and you also opened yourself emotionally by allowing your feelings to get overly or deeply attached.

Let's not forget that you opened yourself spiritually when you made a vow—when the two became one. Shutting down emotionally and cutting off the physical doesn't mean you closed the emotional and spiritual doors. You can shut down emotionally while your emotions remain attached. You can shut down spiritually while your spirit is open to forgiving and rekindling the relationship.

Even though you're not with the other person physically, your mind, will, emotions, memories, imagination, and personality are tied to them. You're committed to the uncommitted. Just because you're not with them doesn't mean you are free from them.

I learned this principle when I got out of prison, and my ex popped in to see me at my grandmother's house, where I was staying at the time. When she knocked on the door and I answered it, my stomach hit the floor as soon as I saw her face. I broke out in a sweat, my heart pounded, and I prayed for strength. Before that day, I hadn't seen her in over four years. Seeing her again awakened old memories.

I was strong, but I didn't know how strong I was—until the end of our eight-hour conversation. She tried to spend the night with me, but I politely declined her request. Did I want her to spend the night? Yes. My flesh tried to rise, but my relationship with God was too strong. Therefore, her invitation into temptation wasn't even a thought in my mind.

Even though we hadn't seen each other, much less been together, in years, the attachment I had for her went from a heavy soul tie to a light soul tie. The tie was still there, but I was in full control.

At the end of our conversation, I learned that I was internally stronger even while being in her physical presence. Yes, I still had a light soul tie because according to 1 Corinthians 6:15-20 (TPT), two people can become one flesh after sexual intercourse. It doesn't matter whether you're married or not; once the sexual union takes place, two can become one mentally, emotionally, and spiritually. Because of our sexual past, I still had some severing to finish. You have to trust that what God doesn't do immediately, He will continue to do progressively.

This is the mystery of soul ties. Ungodly and unhealthy soul ties hinder and stagnate life. One could be further along in life were it not for these soul ties.

Let's take a brief look at how this happens:

- **Ungodly and unhealthy soul ties create dysfunction.** Anytime you live with dysfunction, you have only an illusion of peace but never experience true lasting peace.
- **Ungodly and unhealthy soul ties impede your potential.** Rather than the best coming from you, the worst is.
- **Ungodly and unhealthy soul ties distract you.** The enemy can do this in many ways, but one sure way is to send someone into your life to distract you.
- **Ungodly and unhealthy soul ties can lead you into depression.** When you see that the relationship isn't improving, but your love won't allow you to leave, you'll settle, which can lead to depression because settling is not fulfilling.
- **Ungodly and unhealthy soul ties can turn you into the victim.** Because you believe you can't win in the relationship, you try to get sympathy from others by playing the victim.
- **Ungodly and unhealthy soul ties cause you to live in continual offense.** The person you are in a relationship with hurts you continually, but you can't get free. You will always be subject to offense.
- **Ungodly and unhealthy soul ties create trust issues.** Let's face it, if your partner cheats on you, abuses and disrespects you for years, you're living in dysfunction.

If you ever get free from them, how can you not have trust issues in the next relationship?

- **Ungodly and unhealthy soul ties negate the ability to live a productive life for Christ.** Being in a relationship with someone who is selfish and doesn't live a Christlike life puts you at risk of taking on their characteristics.

- **Ungodly and unhealthy soul ties cloud your judgment.** This making you unable to see life accurately.

- **Ungodly and unhealthy soul ties have the power to make your life a living hell here on Earth.** You are reduced to merely existing, rather than truly living. It's like walking on eggshells to protect yourself from disappointment and living in fear.

- **Ungodly and unhealthy soul ties can be addictive.** If your mate can get you addicted to them, then they'll never worry about you leaving them. The sad thing is that you are committed to your partner, but they are not committed to you, and when you accept this one-way commitment, it becomes the source of their power over you.

I hope you understand the root intents of ungodly and unhealthy soul ties. They have the power to steal your identity. All results are fruit from this root. The root or heart of the enemy's agenda is to steal our identity. If you don't know who you are, then the world, other people, or an ungodly soul tie can turn you into who they want you to be, rather than who God created you to be. From day one, the enemy has always been after our identity—especially the identities of the children of God. One way he does this is by tempting you to enter a relationship in which you become vulnerable to any of the above soul tie consequences. The enemy knows that God the Father has a plan and a purpose for your life. He also knows that once you discover it and begin walking in it, you become a threat to the stability and success of his kingdom. So, his goal is to destroy you before you discover God's plan, which will lead you to your true identity.

Before you received Christ as your personal Lord and Savior, you answered to a name or nickname. On the day you were saved (i.e., born again), your name may not have changed in the natural, but it changed in the spiritual, because anytime your spirit changes, your name changes. Jesus said, *"As many as received Him, to them He gave the power to become the sons of God"* (John 1:12).

We're told in the Bible that whenever people had an encounter with God and gave their lives to him, it was the ending of an old name and the beginning of a new name. For example, after Abram's encounter with God, God changed his name to Abraham. After Jacob's encounter, God renamed him Israel. It was first Sarai before God changed her name to Sarah. It was first Cephas before Jesus renamed him Peter. It was Saul before God changed it to Paul. With your name change comes a change to your identity. Your identity change is the opportunity to see yourself in a greater way and on a higher level. If you see yourself differently, you'll expect, create, and live a different life.

After you come into the family of God, you should be excited to see yourself new because God gives you new honor, new authority, and a new purpose for your new life. The enemy knows that when you see yourself being made new—your new identity in Christ—quite naturally you'll pursue an entirely new life. Truly, your new identity replaces your old identity. Your new identity is based on who God the Father says you are.

When I came into the conviction of my identity in Christ, I investigated the scriptures, so I would be in total alignment with who God the Father was calling me to be, and who God said I am, based on His Word.

The following is what I found about our identity in Christ:

- *"You are a new creation in Christ Jesus."* (2 Corinthians 5:17)
- *"You are God's child that's been born of the incorruptible seed of the Word of God."* (1 Peter 1:23)
- *"You are a partaker of the inheritance of the saints in light."* (Colossians 1:12)
- *"You are the temple of the Holy Spirit."* (1 Corinthians 6:19)
- *"You are blessed."* (Galatians 3:4 and Deuteronomy 28:1-14)
- *"You are the elect of God."* (Colossians 3:12)
- *"You are a royal priesthood; you are chosen; you are a peculiar people."* (1 Peter 2:9)
- *"You are righteous and holy."* (Ephesians 4:24)
- *"You are free from sin."* (Romans 6:18)
- *"You are a saint."* (Ephesians 1:1)
- *"You are a citizen of Heaven."* (Philippians 3:20)
- *"You are the first fruits among His creation."* (James 1:18)
- *"You are an ambassador of Christ."* (2 Corinthians 5:20)
- *"You are God's workmanship, created in Christ Jesus for good works."* (Ephesians 2:10)
- *"You are a partaker of His Divine Nature."* (2 Peter 1:4)
- *"You are sealed with the Holy Spirit of promise."* (Ephesians 1:13)
- *"You are joint heirs with Christ."* (Romans 8:17)
- *"You are more than a conqueror."* (Romans 8:37)

- *"You are dead to sin."* (1 Peter 2:24)
- *"You are strong in the Lord."* (Ephesians 6:10)
- *"You are accepted in the beloved."* (Ephesians 1:6)
- *"You are complete in Him [Christ Jesus]."* (Colossians 2:10)
- *"You are alive with Christ."* (Ephesians 2:5)
- *"You've been crucified with Christ."* (Galatians 2:20)
- *"You are reconciled to God."* (2 Corinthians 5:18)
- *"You are the salt of the Earth, and the light of the world."* (Matthew 5:13-14)
- *"You are the righteousness of God in Christ Jesus."* (2 Corinthians 5:21)
- *"You are the beloved of God."* (Romans 1:7)
- *"God always causes you to triumph."* (2 Corinthians 2:14)
- *"You are seated with Christ Jesus in Heavenly places."* (Ephesians 2:6)
- *"You are God's co-laborer."* (1 Corinthians 3:9)
- *"You are a holy partaker of a Heavenly calling."* (Hebrews 3:1)
- *"You are born of God."* (1 John 5:18)
- *"Nothing can separate you from the Love of God."* (Romans 8:35-38)

These several verses are just a few Scripture references that state who God says you are in Him and His Word. Grab hold of these because when the enemy attempts to get you connected to an ungodly soul tie, or when he tries to turn the healthy soul tie into an unhealthy one, you'll recognize that he's after your identity. You don't have to fall prey to him.

One of the most common ways ungodly and unhealthy soul ties can steal your identity is by a spirit of condemnation. The word "condemnation" means, "to express a strong disapproval of someone." Condemnation is powerful because it creates an intense negative feeling. Feeling as though God or your spouse, parents, friends, siblings, church family, or mate disapproves of you, makes you disapprove of yourself.

In today's culture, a most prevalent lie says, "You are what you feel. You are how you feel, and you are the thing that you feel." If the enemy discovers that you will believe this lie, he tries his best to connect you to an ungodly soul tie that will work on you to accept the spirit of condemnation.

Condemnation produces self-hate, self-rejection, neglect, and abandonment. When those four feelings unite and work together, they produce a spirit of fear. One of the most powerful principles about condemnation is that condemnation is only as powerful as you allow it to be. You don't have to accept condemnation from anyone. You have the choice to accept or reject it.

Understand this: Your friends, coworkers, or mate can express disapproval of you, but it doesn't mean they are correct, and you do not have to accept their disapproval. In other words, you're not powerless. The only way you are powerless to condemnation is when you accept it. The enemy knows that condemnation coming through an ungodly soul tie is hard to reject; disapproval from someone you are in a relationship with is hard to ignore. Remember, how our mates see us influences how we see ourselves. The enemy knows this and uses it to get us to turn away from our God-given identity and accept the identity that others want to assign to us.

Jesus said, *"If thou canst believe, all things are possible to him that believeth"* (Mark 9:23). Here we learn that positive things are possible if we believe. But this truth applies to condemnation too. Believing the condemnation gives it power over you. Likewise, it's possible to untangle the soul tie, and it's possible to stay tied for the rest of your life. Your heart can be made whole, and it's possible to remain broken. It's possible to accept condemnation, and it's also possible to reject condemnation. All things are possible if you believe. Your choice is to believe what God says about you or believe what others say.

Therefore, the most important word in this scripture is "if" because it creates a conditional statement. "If" is the condition that you'll either accept others' disapproval or reject it. This means the condemnation or encouragement is only as powerful as you allow *if* you believe. Religion or relationship is powerful only if you believe. Depression or acceptance is powerful only if you believe. Deliverance and freedom are powerful only if you believe. Self-pity or self-confidence is powerful only if you believe.

This scripture is powerful because Jesus made the playing field level when he said, "all" things are possible if you believe. Satan knows this as he studies us deeply so that when he condemns us, he uses relational condemnation. Since we believers are called to live according to love, acceptance, and trust, what better way to get a believer to accept Satan's condemnation? The enemy leans toward ungodly and unhealthy soul ties because it's an easy avenue to accomplishing his goals. Relational condemnation makes you feel as if you're not good enough or unwanted.

It's dangerous to be connected to someone who you feel like doesn't want you—especially if you want them. You'll try to make them see how much you want them, and it will give them the freedom to treat you however they want to. One day, they may feel like dealing with you, talking to you, or being around you, but the next day, they may feel just the opposite and won't deal with you, talk to you, or be with you. You've given them permission to treat you as they please, including condemning you. Over time, this person will turn you into whatever they want. In other words, they will steal your identity.

When you are connected to an ungodly soul tie, and they don't want you, they will do several things.

Let's take a brief look at these tactics:

1. **They won't pay attention to you because you're not that important to them.** Your presence is according to their whims and desires.
2. **They refuse to pour anything positive into you, if it doesn't benefit them.** The only reason they build you up is for the sole purpose of you building them up.
3. **Their actions and words prove they don't care about your needs.** Your needs are the least of their concern. If you want to be included in their plans, if you want to be known by their family, if you want them to acknowledge your desires, or if you want affection from them, then don't hold your breath, because you're not a priority to them.
4. **They demand that you fulfill their needs.** Being tied to an ungodly soul tie is always about the other person and never about you. They are concerned with what you can give and do for them, while they neglect what you want or need. As soon as you can't fulfill their desires, they threaten to break up with you or leave you. When you can't meet their needs (e.g., financially, sexually, personally, or emotionally), you become useless to them.
5. **They refuse to sacrifice for you.** Most of the time, when you're with them, you must go to the restaurants they choose, take part in the things they want to do,

and attend the events they want to attend. Your suggestions are rarely accepted. If you ask them to come to an event with you or help you with something, then they refuse to sacrifice any plans they might have to attend with you or aid you. They will not come out of their comfort zone to do anything sacrificial for you.

6. **They won't try to see the best in you, but they are quick to point out your every flaw.** Instead of encouraging your strengths, they are quick to tell you what you don't have, and who you're not. When a person only wants you for what you have or can do for them, they'll condemn you for not living up to their selfish expectations.

Relational condemnation is demonstrated when your mate doesn't respect you, and if you've allowed this person to disrespect you for so long, then they believe you don't deserve respect.

The following is a brief rundown of why an ungodly soul tie won't respect you:

1. **You don't have boundaries, so you allow them to get away with anything.** They see you as weak because you don't show them your strength. Anytime you allow a person to abuse you, cheat on you, talk down to you, or not value you, they will consider you to be weak.

2. **They don't see you as a leader but as a follower.** Leaders stand up, create boundaries, and take control of their lives. Followers go along to get along. If you are in a relationship with someone who doesn't have the Spirit of God living in them to convict them of their foul

and evil ways, then they will get away with whatever you allow. This is what a follower does.

3. **They don't think they can learn anything from you.** You may be a lot smarter than they perceive, and they can learn a lot from you, but because they don't respect you, they refuse to listen to you. Therefore, according to them, you are always taking mental and emotional withdrawals from them without making any deposits into them.

4. **They secretly think they are better than you.** A relationship in which the other person thinks that you don't bring anything to the relationship typically means that they think they are better than you, and that you need them. Do they cut you off every time you start speaking? Do they often disregard your suggestions? Do they downplay or minimize your visions and dreams? If you said yes to any of these questions, then that means they have labeled you as "worthless."

5. **They don't think you believe in yourself.** Anytime you're timid around them, they interpret it as you not believing in yourself. In their mind, if you don't believe in yourself, then you shouldn't expect them to believe in you.

6. **They don't respect you because they don't respect themselves.** A person with an apathetic mentality doesn't care about themselves; therefore, they cannot care about you.

The Bible says, *"There is therefore now no condemnation to them which are in Christ Jesus, who walk not after the flesh, but after the Spirit"* (Romans 8:1). This means that at the moment you accept Jesus as your Lord and Savior, condemnation is no longer a part of your identity.

Our goal as Christians is to walk in the Spirit of God and not after the flesh. Whenever we walk in the flesh, we allow the spirit of condemnation to get the best of us. If you choose to go through life with an ungodly soul tie, then you run the risk of changing your identity from a child of God to a victim of the enemy. If the enemy can steal your identity, then it will be extremely easy for him to deter you away from your God-given destiny. Be careful of the spirit of condemnation.

Grasp the truth that as a child of God, you are no longer condemned. This is great news! If God doesn't condemn you, no one has any right to condemn you.

PART THREE
SEVER THE SOUL TIES!

CHAPTER 12

IT'S TIME TO DECLARE WAR!

WE'VE COME a long way on our journey of learning about soul ties. I'm confident you have a thorough understanding of soul ties and covenant connections. You know how to identify heavy soul ties, moderate soul ties, and light soul ties. By now you know which soul ties you want to stay connected to and which ones you're ready to release.

Throughout these chapters, you learned how to identify if you're tied, and how the tie was established. You know the enemy's secrets about ungodly soul ties and learned that what you don't know can keep you tied.

Now it's time for the good part: how to sever the soul tie.

As it pertains to intimate relationships for most people living in western culture, ungodly soul ties are created from the bottom up: from the body to the soul then to the spirit. Two people have sex first (the body). Then they try to figure out what they want to do with their lives both individually and corporately (the soul). Last, they talk about their spiritual beliefs (the spirit).

Most often, two people come together and instantly start performing marital duties (e.g., putting each other's names on their bank accounts). One spouse may allow the other to discipline their children if they have kids. Of course, they move in together, as if they are already spouses. They interact in all these things without ever asking each other, "Where does your faith lie? Do you believe in Jesus?

Western society has led people to believe it's normal to create soul ties from the bottom up. But when you want to sever the soul tie, you must start from the top and move to the bottom.

According to Jesus, words are Spirit: *"The Words that I speak unto you, they are Spirit, and They are Life"* (John 6:63). The law of faith says, *"Before I possess a thing, I must confess a thing."* God the Father operated in the law of faith: *"In the beginning, God created the Heaven and the Earth. The Earth was without form and void, and darkness was upon the face of the deep, and the Spirit of God moved upon the face of the waters, and God said, 'Let there be light,' and there was light"* (Genesis 1:1-3).

Can you see that God the Father had to confess before He possessed? He said, "Let there be light" and there was light. Since you and I are made in the image of God, it's our job to create in the same way he created. He created by way of his words.

One way soul ties are created is by words. Therefore, for a soul tie to be broken, it must be broken by words.

The law of faith is demonstrated in this:

> "But what does it say? The word is near you, in
> your mouth and in your heart [*i.e., the word of
> faith which we preach*], that if you confess with

> your mouth the Lord Jesus and believe in your
> heart that God has raised Him from the dead,
> you will be saved, for with the heart, one
> believes unto righteousness, and with the
> mouth, confession is made unto salvation."

> — ROMANS 10:8-10 (NKJV)

The law of faith is executed when a person receives salvation because you must confess salvation before you can possess it. Therefore, you must apply the law of faith to get into the Kingdom of God. To access anything from the Kingdom of God, you must apply the law of faith. For example, the law of faith is executed in marriage with the phrase *"for better or worse, 'til death do us part."* Two people are vowing to remain as one until death. So, you must confess to possess your marriage.

Deliverance, freedom, joy, peace, wisdom, understanding, knowledge, and supernatural strength are all attributes that come from the kingdom of God. Soul ties are spiritual, so it takes spiritual things to remove a spiritual problem. Once again, you can't repair a spiritual defect with a worldly mindset.

Scripture tells us the weapons of our warfare are not carnal, but it doesn't tell us what the weapons are (2 Corinthians 10:4). May I submit that the weapons of our warfare are words? To sever the soul tie, you must start in the spirit. The tools to maneuver you through the spirit realm are words.

To sever a soul tie, the first step must be accepting Jesus as your personal Lord and Savior. Invite Jesus into your heart.

All you must do is say this prayer aloud right now:

Father, in the name of Jesus, I confess that I am a sinner. And I ask you to forgive me for every sin, every iniquity, every trespass, and every transgression. I repent from all my sinful ways, And I turn to you totally in spirit, soul, and body. On this day, I break the allegiance; I renounce the allegiance, and I renounce the covenant I made with Satan and the kingdom of darkness. I accept Jesus Christ as my Lord and Savior. I believe that Jesus came to the Earth, lived 33 years without sin, and willingly went to the cross. He hung; he bled, and he died for all the sins of humankind, including mine. Three days later, he was resurrected from the grave with all power in His hands. I confess that Jesus Christ is Lord in Heaven and on Earth. I want to receive Jesus Christ as my personal Lord and Savior, And right now, I ask the Holy Spirit of God to come into my heart and make me a new creation.

Holy Spirit of God, you're so welcome to become one with my spirit, regenerate my spirit, and adopt me into the family of God. Holy Spirit of love, come. Holy Spirit of freedom, come. Holy spirit of power, come. Holy Spirit of truth, come.

Father, I thank you for accepting me. I thank you for affirming me. I thank you for adopting me into your family, and I thank you for your patience and mercy you've extended me. I am your son/daughter, and today my life is changed from the inside out.

In Jesus' name,

amen.

If you said this prayer and truly mean it from the bottom of your heart, God the Holy Spirit just moved into your spirit, he eliminated the nature of Satan, and he gave you the nature of Christ.

When you accept Christ, your spirit becomes one with His Spirit: *"He that is joined unto the Lord is one spirit"* (1 Corinthians 6:17); *"As He* [Jesus] *is, so are we in this world"* (1 John 4:17). When one accepts Jesus Christ as Lord and Savior, not only does that person's spirit change from darkness to light, but it also gains the privilege of being empowered by the Holy Spirit as God's child. This is important because your perspective (i.e., how you see yourself) will decide your outcome of receiving healing and wholeness, or you'll stay in dysfunction and brokenness.

On the day you receive Christ Jesus as your Lord and Savior, you no longer must see yourself as a sinner because your position changes to a child of God. Something happens on the inside when you see yourself as perfect in the eyes of God. You may have been told that you will always be a sinner, saved by grace. Honestly, that's an old religious lie. Maybe you have heard it for so long that it has formed a stronghold in your mind. We are saved by grace (Ephesians 2:8), but we are *sons and daughters* who have been saved by grace, not sinners who have been saved by grace.

Remember, if the enemy can steal your identity, then he can also steal your destiny. He wants you to call yourself a "sinner," so you'll give yourself a license to sin when things get hard and so you will give yourself the right to quit when things do not go your way.

Let's say you decide to repent and turn your life around. At that point, you refuse to continue indulging in fornication. As the journey gets strenuous, your desire for fornication strengthens. If you continue to call yourself a sinner, eventually you will be okay with giving up resistance as soon as the thought, "I'm a sinner; nobody is perfect, including me. God knows my heart," enters your mind.

As you begin to sever the soul tie, you will run into hard things. But just because things get hard doesn't mean that the journey is not from God. Seeing yourself the way God sees you is hard. I'm thoroughly convinced and fully persuaded that God sees us from the spirit first.

In Christ, we are righteous. In Christ, we are a new creation. In Christ, we are sons and daughters, and in Christ, we are more than conquerors. If you aren't in Christ, then you'll never be empowered with the Holy Spirit. The Holy Spirit is the One who gives you the spirit of wisdom, knowledge, understanding, truth, vision, forgiveness, power, counsel, peace, freedom, faith, boldness, grace, love, and hope, as well as the Mind of Christ to sever the soul tie.

When the Holy Spirit is in you, He gives you everything you need, anytime you feel like you're in a dark, hopeless place, while you're on the journey to freedom and wholeness. The journey will teach you how to develop, keep, sustain, and maximize a relationship with God the Holy Spirit.

Because soul ties are spiritual, you need the greatest and most powerful Spirit to be on your side and fight on your behalf. According to John 4:24, Jesus said that God is a Spirit. In Matthew 10:20, The Holy Spirit is referred to as the Spirit of the Father. Therefore, it's obvious that the Holy Spirit is the Spirit of God.

The Holy Spirit is a Spirit who has a soul. We see three instances in scripture when the Holy Spirit can be emotional. *"But they rebelled and vexed His Holy Spirit"* (Isaiah 63:10). In

Hebrew, the word "vexed" means "to be distressed, as it pertains to a state of emotional distress, sorrow, and to be filled with pain."

"And grieve not the Holy Spirit of God" (Ephesians 4:30). The Greek word for "grieve" means "to be sad, sorrowful, and distressed."[2] Finally, *"Quench not the Spirit"* (1 Thessalonians 5:19). The Greek word for "quench" means "to extinguish a fire, to stop a fire and to snuff out."[3] This strongly suggests a prophetic enthusiasm of the Holy Spirit.

These verses are imperative to prove this point: You are a spirit-being with a soul, but your spirit and soul live in your body. The Holy Spirit is a Spirit-Being who has a soul, and He wants to live in you, but you must allow Him in.

When you allow the Holy Spirit to come inside you and become one with your spirit, He wants to knit, cleave, and bond with your soul. As you release your mind, you will exchange it for His mind. As you release your will, you exchange it for His will. He will teach you how to release your emotions in exchange for His emotions. You exchange your soul for His soul to the best of your ability.

From there, you'll be thoroughly equipped to sever every ungodly and unhealthy soul tie to which you've ever been connected. Can you imagine the strongholds, lies, memories, and impure imaginations that the Holy Spirit will empower and enable you to eliminate from your mind? Can you imagine the Love of God you'll experience in your heart?

You must be convinced of this: God wants you to be totally healed and made whole from all hurts and pains from the past, present, or future. What better person to heal you, set you free, and make you whole than the Spirit of God, who created you?

The Bible says, *"For what man knoweth the things of a man—save the spirit of man, which is in him? Even so, the things of God knoweth no man, but the Spirit of God"* (1 Corinthians 2:11). The soul tie is a mystery. So why wouldn't a person who has an ungodly or unhealthy soul tie want to employ the manufacturer to aid in breaking the soul tie? Remember, God created soul ties in Genesis 2:24. Therefore, if God created them and the Spirit of God becomes one with you, don't you think He'll teach you how to sever and destroy the ungodly and unhealthy soul ties if He wants you to be free and made whole? Absolutely! Remember, your first step is to receive Jesus Christ as your Lord and Savior. If you have not yet done so, now is the time to go back and pray the prayer of repentance and acceptance.

You will feel peace, love, and joy as well as a sense of weight or heat when the Holy Spirit of God manifests His presence upon you.

Because Christ lives in you, you must honor, value, and esteem two important principles: (1) The God of the entire universe lives in you; nothing that's on the outside of you is bigger than the God who lives in you, and (2) Christ lives in you; therefore, you are now in the family of God. God is fighting for you, and He will empower you with everything you need to win the battle of becoming free from ungodly and unhealthy soul ties.

You can use the name of Jesus, the blood of Jesus, the power of the cross, the finished works of Jesus, the Word of Jesus, and the Spirit of Jesus on your behalf against demons and all of darkness. You can use these in prayer and your declarations. Now you have all the power and assistance from heaven, so you can be delivered and walk in total freedom.

THE POWER OF PRAYER

Most people believe that prayer is simply a nice gesture. However, to the children of God, prayer is one of the spiritual weapons we use to destroy the works, lies, and powers of darkness. Prayer is the heartbeat of your spiritual life. Prayer is to your spirit what your heart is to your body. You can't have a healthy body if you don't have a healthy heart. Similarly, you can't have a healthy spirit if you don't have a healthy prayer life.

As children of God, we don't pray with the sole motive of getting something from God; rather, we pray to connect to God. Plus, we strive daily to become someone new in God. The priority of prayer is not always designed to bless you but to change you. Prayer is not only coming to God and telling him everything you want or need but also waiting until God speaks to you. When He speaks to you, what He says will change you.

Anytime you approach God the Father in prayer, start with adoration, which is giving God the utmost esteem, love, respect, and reverence by paying divine honor to God. This is expressed when you approach God the Father by acknowledging him by name. Next, ask Him to fill your atmosphere with the presence of the Holy Spirit. You can call on the names of the Father, the names of the Holy Spirit, and the names of Jesus. You can't show adoration if you don't know His names.

Let's briefly mention the names of Jesus, the Holy Spirit, and God, starting with Jesus:

- *Wonderful, Counselor, Mighty God, Everlasting Father, and the Prince of Peace*
- *Alpha and the Omega, the Almighty*

- *Beloved*
- *Christ*
- *Chief Cornerstone*
- *Door to the Sheep*
- *Faithful and True*
- *Holy One*
- *Just*
- *King*
- *Lion*
- *Lamb*
- *Mediator of the New Covenant*
- *Messiah*
- *Nazarene*
- *Redeemer*
- *Resurrection*
- *Savior*
- *Servant*
- *Son of God*
- *Tried and Tested*
- *The Word*
- *Wisdom of God*

In the Scriptures, the Holy Spirit is referred to as the following:

- *Spirit of Jesus*
- *Spirit of the Father*
- *Spirit of God*
- *Breath of Life*
- *Spirit of the Lord*
- *Spirit of Wisdom*
- *Spirit of Understanding*
- *Spirit of Might*
- *Spirit of Counsel*

- *Spirit of Knowledge*
- *Spirit of Freedom*
- *Spirit of Love*
- *Spirit of Joy*
- *Spirit of Truth*
- *Spirit of Comfort*
- *Spirit of Power*

God the Father is known as the following:

- *Abba*
- *Ancient of Days*
- *Most High God*
- *Father*
- *Elohim*
- *El-Shaddai*
- *Yahweh*
- *Jehovah*
- *Jehovah Jireh*
- *Jehovah Nissi*
- *Jehovah Shalom*
- *God of Abraham, Isaac, and Jacob*
- *Father of Glory*
- *Father of Lights*
- *Eternal*
- *Only Wise God*
- *Shield*
- *Strong Tower*

Knowing these names will aid you in severing soul ties. There will be times when you will have to choose to either magnify the pain you're feeling, or the name of the Lord to experience the peace of, in, and with God.

Before you pray, it's wise to bring God into the scene so you can get into His presence. *"Where the Spirit of the Lord is, there is liberty"* (2 Corinthians 3:17). I'm sure you'll go through moments of loneliness, and you will be heavily tempted to call the person who broke your heart or hurt you. You'll be tempted to ask them to comfort you, even though you know that their presence is only going to rekindle a fire that you're so desperately trying to put out.

Therefore, if you ask the Holy Spirit of God to come onto the scene and be present with you, He will come and give you the peace, strength, and comfort you need to make it through those hard moments. This is not religious prayer but relational prayer.

Because the priority of prayer is to change you, don't just leave after you have told God everything you want to say. Instead, wait to hear what God wants to say to you. The voice of God comes through spontaneous thoughts that grab your attention and produce joy, excitement, peace, hope, love, and life. When God the Father speaks, His voice will change you by what He says, while also bringing a heavenly blessing to you.

When I was going through the process of severing the soul tie from my ex-girlfriend, the pain, hurt, embarrassment, and loneliness caused me to develop a consistent prayer life. When I prayed and received peace after the first experience, I continued praying to receive comfort and assurance. I got tired of taking my pain to so-called friends. I got tired of telling anybody who would listen about how hurt I was. I felt like I needed someone to listen to me.

Eventually, I discovered there weren't many people who had the wisdom to help me get free from the pain. They felt sorry for me, but they couldn't help me or deliver me. One day, a great friend of mine spoke words that changed my entire outlook and approach to the pain. He said, "James, I want to say something to you as a friend, and I hope you can receive this in the right way."

"Okay. I can receive it," I said.

"Man, you should be tired of running around telling all these guys about how hurt you are and about how bad your girl dogged you out. You're not the only person whose heart has been broken, and you won't be the last. You say you are a believer, so instead of running around telling these dudes about everything you're going through with your girl, when are you going to start praying and telling God about it?"

"Bro! You don't think I pray? I tell God about it all the time!"

"I'm sure you pray and tell God about your problems and your troubles, and I'm sure you haven't thought about waiting on Him to answer you after you finish praying, but you haven't grown up and matured to the point of telling God how big He is in your life! If you want some advice and wisdom on how to deal with this, then get some Heavenly wisdom and stop searching for earthly wisdom. Heavenly wisdom will heal you and build you, but earthly wisdom will feel sorry for you and talk about you to other people as soon as you leave their presence."

That conversation changed my approach to prayer, it changed my mind about prayer, it changed my expectations about prayer, and it changed my prayer life. The next prayer I prayed, I followed his instructions, and the peace of God started flooding my life. I must admit, my friend was an angel sent from heaven to lead me to discover the power of prayer as I started severing the soul tie.

Adoration is so powerful because it teaches you how to get your eyes off the pain, hurt, and problems; then it instructs you to place your focus on how big your God is.

The God of the universe, whom you are praying to, lives inside you. Part of your prayer must include thanksgiving, which is so powerful because you're not focused on what you don't have, and you become grateful for what you do have. You may be hurting, but you still have breath in your lungs. You may be lonely, but you haven't lost your mind. You might be embarrassed, but you still have your health and strength. You might be broken, but you still have the God of the universe living inside you. Hope is waiting on you to receive it if only you believe.

In your private time of prayer, worship is also a powerful weapon. During your time of worship, you must remain focused. Worship is not listening to songs that magnify your struggles and pain; rather, worship is an opportunity to lift God the Father, Son, and Holy Spirit above everything you're going through.

In worship, the words lead you into mentally picturing your freedom, peace, strength, and new life. You must remain focused because whatever you keep beholding (mentally picturing) is what you'll become. Therefore, in times of worship, keep your eyes closed, then ask Holy Spirit to release the love of God fresh on you and to renew every part of you. If you don't sense it happening, imagine the love of God falling fresh and renewing every part of you.

Confession is the next part of prayer. Confess any known or unknown sin. Acknowledge things like unforgiveness, bitterness, rage, hatred, or envy. During your intimate prayer time, give up your right to hold onto anything that can create a blockage in your heart. Jesus said, *"Therefore, if thou bring thy gift to the altar, and there rememberest that thy brother hath ought against thee, leave there thy gift before the altar and go thy way; first, be reconciled to thy brother, and then come offer thy gift"* (Matthew 5:23-24). In other words, as children of God, we should resolve our issues.

The first step is to admit or confess them before we come to God in prayer: *"If a man says, 'I love God,' and hateth his brother, he is a liar, for how can he that loveth not his brother, whom he hath seen, love God, whom he hath not seen? And this commandment have we from him, that he who loveth God love his brother also"* (1 John 4:20-21).

When you admit, confess, and try to resolve your struggles before you ask God for anything in prayer, it gives the Holy Spirit permission to cleanse you and empower you (1 John 1:9) with whatever you need to overcome the struggle.

After confession comes repentance, telling God the Father that it's your most sincere desire to turn away from anything you're struggling with and to embrace His will, His way, and His love.

Repentance isn't *"I'm sorry for what I've done;"* that's remorse. Remorse is a small part of repentance, but repentance means "to turn away and change your mind from unrighteousness to righteousness."[4] Repentance isn't authentic until your mind is changed. I know plenty of people who are remorseful because they disobeyed the Voice of God, but they are not remorseful to the point of hating their disobedience.

For example, a husband taking part in sinful and adulterous ways will be remorseful because his wife caught him, and he doesn't want to lose his family. Furthermore, she will never know if he repents (i.e., changes his mind) until she sees his disdain for the spirit that tempted and drove him into adultery.

At this point, she's forced to monitor his actions, maturity, and growth. All she can do is pray until she sees the fruits of repentance in his life. Once the decision to repent is cemented in your heart, it's time to renounce the agreement, allegiance, attachment, and covenant you made with the person you formed a soul tie with.

Not only must he renounce these things but also the spirit he succumbed to. The word "renounce" means "(1) to formally declare one's abandonment of a claim, right, or possession; (2) to give up, refuse, or resign, usually by formal declaration; (3) to refuse to follow, obey, or recognize any further; (4) to officially give up or turn away from." An example of this is found in 1 Peter 2:1: *"Therefore, laying aside all malice, all deceit, hypocrisy, envy, and all evil speaking"* (NKJV).

After you've been heartbroken by an ungodly soul tie, many forms of evil may linger in your heart. The same way you created the emotional attachments by way of a spoken vow is the same way you'll destroy the emotional attachments: by renouncing the vow. Sometimes the tie can be so strong you will find yourself renouncing it every day. This is okay because you are renewing your mind to the truth of your decision instead of succumbing to hurtful feelings (we will discuss this in the next chapter).

If you're divorced, you've accepted it, and you're ready to move forward with your life, you still must renounce the covenant, allegiance, agreement, and attachment you made with your former spouse. You created the cleaving, binding, and knitting together of your souls by words. Now you must use the power of your spoken words to renounce your vow. (This is a mystery of spiritual soul ties.)

Last, after your renouncement, command any spirits to leave your body in the name of Jesus. Depending on how heavy the tie was and how long your heart was broken, a spirit of trauma may linger in your soul. Use the name of Jesus and command the spirit of trauma to leave every dimension of your soul and body.

This also goes for the spirits of brokenness, hate, envy, rejection, neglect, unworthiness, anxiety, guilt, shame, animosity, fear, bitterness, condemnation, resentment, greed, perversion, and any other spirits that may have come with the person you had an ungodly or unhealthy soul tie with. These things could have remained with you.

When you become connected with another person, you become one with them during the union. When you separate, you each take a part of the other's heart and soul with you.

In the name of Jesus, call back every righteous part of you that they took. Call your strength back. Call your peace of mind back. Call your mind, purpose, faith, and life back. If you got so deep into them that you lost the greatest parts of who you were (e.g., your identity), then you now have the authority in the name of Jesus Christ to call back every God-given quality that God the Father created you with. God never intended you to give away the peace He gave you, and now that you are in the Family of God, you've been gifted with the authority to call back the Heavenly qualities that the enemy stole from you during that union.

Prayer's role in severing the soul tie is that if you don't pray and ask Heaven to get involved on your behalf, then Heaven cannot and will not act—until you ask. In Genesis 1:26, God's original mandate and purpose for humankind were to *"let them have dominion."* God, in His sovereignty (i.e., supreme reign), transferred the authority and dominion to humankind to govern and reign on Earth. When Adam named the animals and cultivated the Garden of Eden, he was exercising the dominion mandate that God had placed upon his life. He was being a good steward over the assignment that God had entrusted him with. The word "stewardship" means "to be an effective manager over another one's property." In other words, God the Father owned Planet Earth, but He gave Adam and Eve the responsibility to manage, govern, and rule His world. The only way God could get involved was if Adam called upon God in prayer and asked Him to get involved in any of his affairs on Earth. God the Father couldn't just take over—even though it was His—because God said, *"let them."*

God the Father cannot go against His word. He said, *"For you have magnified your word above all your name"* (Psalms 138:2 [NKJV]). This is why Adam used to walk with God in the cool of the day to fellowship with Him in a divine relationship. I'm sure if Adam had any problems too big to manage, then God the Father would have given him the wisdom to manage those problems, or Adam would have invited Him in to take care of those problems. That's exactly what prayer is: inviting God to come into your situation and giving Him the right to reign in and over that situation. When Adam sinned, he transferred his rights of dominion over to Satan, thus Adam became a victim to sin and the nature of sin.

This is why Jesus came to the Earth as a man, walked 33 years without sin, and fulfilled the 613 Laws of Moses and the 10 Commandments. Then He experienced crucifixion, death, and going to hell to destroy it, along with death and the grave. That was Jesus, the sin-offering for all humankind, but that wasn't the end. He was resurrected from the grave because death couldn't hold Him. When God the Father accepted Jesus' sinless blood-sacrifice as the proper payment for sin, Jesus took all the power back into His hands: *"All power is given unto Me in Heaven and Earth. Go ye, therefore, and teach all nations, baptizing them in the name of the Father, and of the Son, and of the Holy Ghost, teaching them to observe all things whatsoever I have commanded you, and, lo, I am with you always—even unto the end of the world"* (Matthew 28:18). This verse is Jesus restoring the power of prayer and authority to the children of God. All we must do is accept Jesus as our Lord and Savior, then our authority in prayer goes into effect.

How could Jesus commission His disciples to go if He didn't have all power and if He wouldn't be with them? Even though our rights and authority have been restored because we have accepted Jesus as Lord and Savior, if we don't pray and ask heaven to come to sever the soul tie, neither the Holy Spirit nor angelic assistance will move until we invite them in prayer.

Another role that prayer plays in severing the soul tie is that if you don't bind it, then Heaven won't bind it either, and if you don't set it loose, then Heaven won't set it loose either. In Matthew 16, the Apostle Peter declared that Jesus was the Christ, the Son of the Living God, before Jesus had revealed Himself as the Messiah.

Peter's revelation and declaration caused Jesus to release a power principle of prayer:

> "And Jesus answered and said unto him, 'Blessed
> art thou, Simon Barjona, for flesh and blood
> hath not revealed it unto thee, but My Father,
> which is in Heaven, and I say also unto thee

that thou art Peter, and upon this rock, I will
build my church, and the gates of hell shall not
prevail against it, and I will give unto thee the
keys of the Kingdom of Heaven, and whatsoever thou shalt bind on Earth shall be bound
in Heaven, and whatsoever thou shalt set
loose on Earth shall be set loose in Heaven."

— MATTHEW 16:17-19

Here's the point: Jesus has become your Lord and Savior; therefore, He gave you the Keys to the Kingdom. According to Jesus,
the Keys of the Kingdom are words. Jesus gave us the power to
bind and set loose when He said, *"Whatsoever you bind on Earth,
it shall be bound on Earth."* The word "whatsoever" in this text
means "whatever." Specific to our topic, "whatever" can refer
not only to ungodly soul ties but also to the spirits of loneliness,
fear, unworthiness, or rejection.

The word "bind" means "to forbid by an indisputable authority." In other words, it's in your power to forbid anything that
hinders your healing or wholeness. If you don't bind it, then it
will not be bound. The term "set loose" means, "to permit by an
indisputable authority."[8] As a child of God, you have the
authority to set loose and bind. If you don't set loose your freedom, joy, and peace, and the Presence of God, then don't expect
any of these Heavenly attributes to flow in your direction.

The role that prayer plays in severing the soul tie depends on
your act of binding every ungodly and unhealthy soul tie that
prevents you from receiving wholeness and healing. Don't forget
that after you bind the darkness, you must also set loose the light.

Another role prayer plays, as it pertains to severing the soul tie, is to give God his rightful position to sit on the throne of your heart. God gets first place back in your life. One of the religious scholars posed a question to Jesus: *"Teacher, which is the greatest commandment in the law?"* (Matthew 22:36 [NKJV]). Jesus pulled from Exodus 20:3, *"Thou shalt have no other gods before Me,"* when he answered him that the greatest command was to love the Lord God with all your heart, all your mind, and all your body.

One of the biggest mistakes many people make, consciously or subconsciously, is to make their relationships, their spouses, or their mates their gods. Anything that takes the number one place in one's life is their god.

This happened to me. I learned a valuable and painful lesson from the experience. Anytime you prioritize anyone or anything above God, it becomes an enemy of God. God is a jealous God, and we were created to worship the Creator, not his creation. Therefore, in prayer, God will inform you that it's time for you to pull down the idol so you can give Him, His rightful place in your life.

Severing the soul tie is the opportunity to receive wisdom in prayer from God. There is a major difference between wisdom from God and good advice from a counselor, therapist, spiritual advisor, relationship coach, best friend, or wise family member. They all could have your best interest at heart and want to help you make the best decisions, but it's dangerous to accept life-changing advice from someone before you go to God first. Good advice comes from the Earth, while Godly wisdom comes from Heaven. Good advice is what others think you should do in your situation, but Godly wisdom is what God has determined for your purpose, destiny, and legacy. Which one do you want?

In prayer, God will speak. His words will change your mind, your approach, and your pursuit of life. After He speaks, if you're still wrestling with what He said, He will confirm His Word in the mouth of your spiritual advisor, counselor, therapist, relationship coach, best friend, or wise family member.

Godly wisdom is vital because everyone's situation and life direction is different from yours. Even though your best friend may be going through a divorce, just as you are, God may give your best friend peace to allow their spouse to go with the divorce and not fight against them, but God may instead tell you to keep praying for your spouse and not to sign any divorce papers because God knows that the plans He has for you and your best friend are different. Before you close this book shut because I made that statement, just hear me out. Sometimes when the abuse is getting ready to lead to a physical death, I personally don't believe God wants you to stay in a marriage until your spouse kills you. Sometimes when the adultery is getting ready to lead to you contracting a deadly sexual transmitted disease, I personally do not believe that God wants you to stay in the marriage until you get infected and eventually die. Can I continue?

Trust that He knows what's best for you. This is why prayer is so important. You need to know what God wants you to do.

This applies to single people also. My wife and I have a story we often tell single people. In the first stages of our dating life, I was still entertaining this one young lady on social media. At the time, all my inbox messages were coming to my laptop computer. One day, my future wife was using it when a message arrived. She opened it and read it. 20 minutes later, she told me that she was done, and our relationship was over. I apologized, but she left. Her past life experience caused her first response to give up, but she knew that she needed God's wisdom. She took the situation and her feelings to God in prayer. He told her to stay. Since that day, we've had no problems, and we've been happily married for six years, with plenty of fruit to show for it. What if my wife had listened to her feelings, rather than what God told her?

In prayer, give God your pain in exchange for his peace. The only prescription for a broken heart diagnosis is the Spirit of God. When the pain seems unbearable, God the Holy Spirit is the only One who is equipped to perform open-heart surgery to heal your broken heart. Usually, this is the place where God the Father receives your invitation to start a daily relationship with Him.

As I was going through a heartbreak and total brokenness for a season. I didn't get much peace from talking to people about the pain I was feeling because all I was doing was venting. The only time I experienced peace was when I was focused on reading the Word of God and when I was in the presence of God. According to Jesus, the Word of God is Spirit and life (John 6:63). Therefore, whenever I received his words (by reading the Bible), I could feel the Word filling up every empty part of my heart. It was repairing every broken piece of my heart.

One day I was sitting on my bed reading the Bible, but it felt like I had a golf ball stuck in my throat. At that moment, I didn't know I was having an anxiety attack. I was under so much pressure because of the heartbreak, I couldn't breathe. As I was reading the Word, I got to Mark chapter 9. This tells of a time when the disciples could not cast the demon out of the boy, so the father brought his child to Jesus. As I read that story, a fleeting thought came to mind: *Tell the spirit of anxiety to leave, in the name of Jesus.*

I thought about this, and then remembered that the night before, I'd had a dream in which demons were choking me and trying to kill me in my sleep. In my dream, as soon as I thought, *"In the Name of Jesus,"* the demons fell to the ground.

So, after contemplating this for a short time, I thought, *"What do I have to lose? I might as well say it—especially if it will relieve this pressure that I am under."*

I said aloud, "In the name of Jesus, I command every evil spirit of anxiety to leave my body."

Instantly the pressure in my throat subsided, and I felt a blanket of peace covering me, from the top of my head to the soles of my feet. From that day forward, anytime I started feeling mental, emotional, or physical pressure come upon me, I opened my mouth and said, "In the name of Jesus, I command every evil spirit to leave my body!" Guess what? The results were the same. The peace of God would flood my body every time. I learned this principle: peace is the manifestation to let you know that you are in the atmosphere of heaven.

Every day, I felt the heaviness from the ungodly soul tie getting lighter and lighter.

Here are three prayers that I encourage you to learn, pray, memorize, and speak aloud, as you're going through the process of severing the ungodly soul tie:

PRAYER #1

FATHER, IN THE NAME OF JESUS. I ACKNOWLEDGE JESUS CHRIST AS MY LORD AND SAVIOR IN EVERY AREA OF MY LIFE. FORGIVE ME FOR EVERY SIN, EVERY STRUGGLE, EVERY INIQUITY, EVERY IDOL, EVERY TRESPASS, AND EVERY TRANSGRESSION. CREATE IN ME A CLEAN HEART AND RENEW WITHIN ME A RIGHT SPIRIT. FATHER, RENEW WITHIN ME A SPIRIT OF LOVE. IN THE NAME OF JESUS, I WANT TO FORGIVE (SAY THE PERSON'S NAME) FOR THE HURT, HEARTBREAK, PAIN, AND BETRAYAL THAT THEY PUT ME THROUGH. IN THE NAME OF JESUS, I RENOUNCE THE SPIRIT OF OFFENSE. I RENOUNCE THE SPIRIT OF UNFORGIVENESS, I RENOUNCE THE SPIRIT OF TRAUMA, I RENOUNCE THE SPIRIT OF ENVY, AND I RENOUNCE THE SPIRIT OF SHAME THAT I'VE BEEN WRESTLING WITH.

IN THE NAME OF JESUS, I FORGIVE MYSELF FOR COMMITTING THE SIN OF FORNICATION, AND I FORGIVE MYSELF FOR CREATING AN UNGODLY SOUL TIE BY WAY OF A VERBAL VOW AND UNHOLY SEXUAL INTERCOURSE. IN THE NAME OF JESUS, AND BY THE AUTHORITY OF JESUS CHRIST, I PLEAD THE BLOOD OF JESUS TO COME BETWEEN ME AND [SAY THE PERSON'S NAME]. IN THE NAME OF JESUS, I PLEAD THE BLOOD OF JESUS OVER THIS UNGODLY, ONE-FLESH UNION. I COMMAND THAT THIS ONE-FLESH UNION BE SEPARATED BY THE AUTHORITY OF JESUS CHRIST. I SEND BACK TO [SAY THE PERSON'S NAME] EVERYTHING I HAVE TAKEN FROM THEM WHEN WE BECAME ONE FLESH. IN THE NAME OF JESUS, AND BY THE BLOOD OF JESUS, I CALL BACK TO ME EVERYTHING THAT I GAVE TO [SAY THE PERSON'S NAME] IN THIS ONE-FLESH UNION. I CALL MY PEACE BACK! I CALL MY JOY BACK! I CALL MY PURPOSE BACK! I CALL MY STRENGTH BACK! I CALL MY PASSION BACK, AND I CALL MY LIFE BACK! IN THE NAME OF JESUS, I RENOUNCE THIS ONE-FLESH UNION WITH [SAY THE PERSON'S NAME]. IN THE NAME OF JESUS, AND BY THE BLOOD OF JESUS, I BREAK THE VOW, AND I ANNUL THE COVENANT THAT I

MADE IN THIS ONE-FLESH UNION. I DECLARE THAT THE BLOOD OF JESUS AND THE POWER OF THE CROSS OF JESUS CHRIST BE A WALL OF SEPARATION BETWEEN ME AND [SAY THE PERSON'S NAME].

IN THE NAME OF JESUS, I SET LOOSE THE HOLY SPIRIT OF FREEDOM. HOLY SPIRIT OF FREEDOM, FALL FRESH UPON ME! IN THE NAME OF JESUS, I SET LOOSE THE HOLY SPIRIT OF LOVE. HOLY SPIRIT OF LOVE, FALL FRESH UPON ME! IN THE NAME OF JESUS, I SET LOOSE THE HOLY SPIRIT OF RESTORATION. HOLY SPIRIT OF RESTORATION, FALL FRESH UPON ME! IN THE NAME OF JESUS, I SET LOOSE THE HOLY SPIRIT OF MIGHT. HOLY SPIRIT OF MIGHT, FALL FRESH UPON ME! IN JESUS' NAME, I WELCOME THE HOLY SPIRIT OF PEACE TO FILL EVERY DIMENSION OF THIS ATMOSPHERE. HOLY SPIRIT OF PEACE, YOU'RE WELCOME TO FLOW IN ME AND COME UPON ME!

IN JESUS' NAME,

AMEN.

PRAYER #2

FATHER, IN THE NAME OF JESUS, I COMMIT ALL MY FACULTIES—SPIRIT, SOUL, AND BODY—TO THE FULLNESS OF JESUS CHRIST. FORGIVE ME FOR MAGNIFYING MY PROBLEMS MORE THAN I MAGNIFY THE NAME OF JESUS! RIGHT NOW, I STEP INTO MY GOD-GIVEN AUTHORITY TO DEMOLISH EVERY FORM OF DARKNESS THAT'S TRYING TO ATTACH ITSELF TO MY LIFE. IN THE NAME OF JESUS, BY THE BLOOD OF JESUS, AND BY THE POWER OF THE CROSS OF JESUS CHRIST, I BIND EVERY ATTACHMENT AND EVERY DESIRE OF LUST, PERVERSION, IMPURE THOUGHTS, SEXUAL IMMORALITY, AND SEXUAL DEPRAVITY. I BREAK THE POWERS OF DARKNESS, AND I SET LOOSE THE KINGDOM OF LIGHT ON MY BEHALF! IN JESUS' NAME, I COMMAND EVERY ILLEGAL AND UNGODLY SPIRIT OF LUST, PERVERSION, DECEIT, AND GREED TO LEAVE MY BODY! I SEND THEM BACK TO

THE PITS OF HELL, AND I REST IN THE PEACE OF GOD. IN THE NAME OF JESUS, I SET LOOSE THE SPIRIT OF GODLY PURITY! IN THE NAME OF JESUS, I SET LOOSE HEAVENLY RIGHTEOUSNESS AND HEAVENLY SANCTIFICATION OVER MY SPIRIT, SOUL, AND BODY. CREATE IN ME A CLEAN HEART AND RENEW WITHIN ME A RIGHT SPIRIT.

HOLY SPIRIT, YOU HAVE THE RIGHT TO CONVICT ME WITH YOUR WORD AND REMIND ME THAT I AM NOT POWERLESS AND THAT I AM THE RIGHTEOUSNESS OF GOD IN CHRIST JESUS. I ACKNOWLEDGE THE FEELINGS OF LONELINESS, FEAR, AND SHAME AND I COMMIT MY MIND, MY IMAGINATIONS, AND MY EMOTIONS TO THE TRUTH OF YOUR WORD. YOUR WORD SAYS THAT I AM MORE THAN A CONQUEROR AND I CAN DO ALL THINGS THROUGH CHRIST WHO STRENGTHENS ME. I CONFESS THAT GREATER IS HE THAT IS IN ME THAN HE THAT IS IN THE WORLD.

FATHER, YOU SAID THAT YOU ARE MY HIDING PLACE, THAT YOU WILL PROTECT ME FROM TROUBLE, AND THAT YOU WILL SURROUND ME WITH SONGS OF DELIVERANCE. THANK YOU FOR ANOINTING ME WITH THE SAME POWER YOU ANOINTED JESUS, TO BE FREE FROM EVERY SPIRIT OF OPPRESSION. IN JESUS' NAME, I BREAK EVERY UNGODLY SOUL TIE, AND I BREAK EVERY UNHEALTHY SOUL TIE FROM EVERY DIMENSION OF MY LIFE. IN THE NAME OF JESUS, I RENOUNCE THE PAST HURTS, BETRAYALS, AND TRAUMA. I LET THEM GO AND CHOOSE TO MOVE FORWARD. I REACH TOWARD THE MARK OF THE PRIZE OF THE HIGH CALLING THAT GOD HAS FOR MY LIFE.

THANK YOU, HOLY SPIRIT, FOR LEADING ME, GUIDING ME, AND EMPOWERING ME TO LIVE A LIFE OF FREEDOM. HOLY SPIRIT OF FREEDOM! I GIVE YOU THE RIGHT TO OPEN MY EYES, UNTIE MY SOUL, AND SET ME FREE FROM EVERY UNGODLY SOUL TIE.

IN JESUS' NAME,

AMEN.

PRAYER #3

Lord Jesus, I believe that you are the Son of God And I'm thoroughly convinced and fully persuaded that you are the only way to God the Father. First, I confess any known sin that I committed, that any of my ancestors or any of my family members committed. I confess every work on the flesh that I've manifested in my past. Lord, I thank you, and I know that you have forgiven me for every sin I've confessed.

And now, Lord, I want to forgive every person who has harmed me, betrayed me, broken me, or wronged me, I forgive them all right now, just as I want you to forgive me. In particular, I forgive (Say the person's name). Right now, in the mighty name of Jesus Christ, I renounce any contact by myself or any of my family members. I renounce any contract, any allegiances, or any covenants that I've made knowingly or unknowingly with Satan, or any occult powers in any form or any kind of secret society. Also, Lord, I commit myself to remove from my house any objects that cause me to be reconnected to an ungodly soul tie. With your help of awareness, I will remove them all.

And now, Lord Jesus, I thank you even more that, on the cross, you were made a curse for me that I might be redeemed from the curse and the receive a blessing. And because of what you did for me on the cross, I now release myself from every ungodly soul tie, from every unhealthy soul tie, from every deserved curse, from every cast curse, from every word curse, from every generational curse, and from every curse that's been tied to my earthly father's and earthly mother's bloodlines. I release myself from every

EVIL INFLUENCE AND EVERY DARK SHADOW OVER ME AND MY FAMILY, WHATEVER SOURCE THEY MAY COME FROM.

I RELEASE MYSELF NOW, IN THE NAME OF JESUS CHRIST OF NAZARETH, FROM EVERY UNGODLY SOUL TIE. LORD, YOU SAID THAT WHOM THE SON HAS SET FREE IS FREE INDEED. I THANK YOU, LORD, THAT I'VE BEEN SET FREE IN YOU AND THROUGH YOU FROM EVERY UNGODLY AND UNHEALTHY SOUL TIE. IN THE NAME OF JESUS, I ASK THE HOLY SPIRIT OF FREEDOM TO FALL FRESH ON ME. HOLY SPIRIT OF LOVE, YOU'RE FREE TO FALL FRESH ON ME. HOLY SPIRIT OF PEACE, YOU'RE WELCOME TO FALL FRESH ON ME. HOLY SPIRIT OF TRUTH, YOU'RE WELCOME TO FALL FRESH ON ME.

IN JESUS' NAME,

AMEN.

CHAPTER 13
I DECLARE WAR!

WHEN SEVERING an ungodly soul tie or dismantling a covenant connection, the most important thing a person can do is evaluate the decision, count the cost of the process, then commit to either severing the soul tie or remain a victim to an ungodly or dysfunctional relationship. This is so important because, for most people who are in a dysfunctional or an ungodly relationship, they truly don't want to sever the soul tie. But they will act as if they do in hopes that their partner will respond and change their ways, thus setting the dysfunctional relationship on the right track.

This evaluation is important because when you decide to sever a soul tie, you cannot give yourself any excuses. You must follow the instructions you received from praying to disconnect from and destroy the covenant with an ungodly soul tie. Your old feelings and emotions will become an enemy to the new instructions, decisions, actions, and habits that you will begin to develop.

The major cost of severing the soul tie is your old experiences and old expectations. If you're not willing to give up the old life, you cannot position yourself for a new life. When you honestly count the cost and understand all that you must give up, you will make your statement a conviction: "I declare war!"

The battlefield is in your mind. The words you hear, the thoughts you entertain, the memories you meditate on, the imagination you feed, the beliefs you receive, and the convictions you accept from this day forward will determine if you will be a victim or come out victorious. The physical relationship you had with the other person is over, but the mental and emotional relationship is ongoing because you haven't declared war against those attachments with that person.

This war is geared toward destroying all thoughts, old memories, impure imaginations, old covenants, old agreements, old beliefs, old convictions, old affections, old feelings, and old allegiances that led you to the ungodly soul tie. Therefore, when you declare war, you are saying, "I'm not giving myself an excuse to accept the abuse [or fill in the blank with the issues], and I am going to take back my life by any means necessary." When you say this to yourself and believe it, you're deciding to love yourself instead of continuing to lose yourself to a person who's done with you or doesn't want you. Then you'll be willing and ready not just to declare war but to start fighting against your internal enemies.

STRATEGY! AGENDA! WEAPONS!

Anytime you declare war against an ungodly soul tie, you need a strategy, an agenda, and weapons. Your strategy is to follow each instruction in this book, starting first with accepting Jesus as your Lord and Savior and then developing your prayer life.

The agenda is to eliminate and eradicate the other person's soul from you, which depends heavily upon your full commitment to the strategy. God's job is to do what you can't do, but he will never do what you are responsible for doing. In other words, God will heal, restore, and make your spirit whole, but you must renew, realign, and reconstruct your soul.

THE STRATEGY: NO CONTACT!

Your first strategy is no contact with that person. If your goal is to sever the soul tie, be delivered from that person, and experience total freedom, you must begin with eliminating every form of physical, mental, and verbal connection. The Bible says, *"So above all, guard the affections of your heart, for they affect all that you are. Pay attention to the welfare of your innermost being, for from there flows the wellspring of life"* (Proverbs 4:23 [TPT]). "Above all" means the number one priority of taking care of yourself starts with guarding the affections of your heart.

Affections are the gentle feelings of liking and caring for someone or something. However, love is deeper and stronger than affection. Love starts with a decision and then develops stronger and deeper feelings. I am telling you so you won't continue to believe the lie that will keep you tied to an ungodly soul tie. Many people claim that we can't help who we fall in love with. If that statement is true, then we must not have any control over our decisions or feelings. That's a lie, because the Word of God commands, *"If you live without restraint and are unable to control your temper, you're as helpless as a city with broken-down defenses, open to attack"* (Proverbs 25:28 [TPT]).

Maybe it feels like you can't control who you fall in love with once you've fallen deeply in love with someone. But before you fell, you decided to allow your affections and feelings to get attached to that person. What if I told you that your feelings can lie to you? If you decided to allow yourself to get deeply connected to a person, right now you can decide to disconnect from that person. I'm not saying that your feelings will change automatically after you decide to disconnect; however, I am saying that when you commit to "no contact," your commitment will strengthen those feelings associated with your decision to sever the soul tie.

No contact strategy is your invitation to begin a detox or a fast. A detox is "a process or period of time in which one abstains from or rids the body of toxic or unhealthy substances."[1] Fasting is the "intentional abstinence of physical gratification to produce spiritual freedom."[2] When a child of God agrees to fast, they deny their fleshly appetites to gain a response from God.

People fast to produce a spiritual breakthrough that will produce emotional freedom, relational freedom, directional freedom, and physical freedom. The purpose of fasting is to get heaven's attention not by what you say but by what you are willing to sacrifice, release, and resist. When you eliminate unhealthy food from your diet for a length of time, your mental and spiritual faculties become uncluttered, allowing you to think and perceive more clearly. When you separate from the ungodly and unhealthy soul ties, your spirit and soul become more sensitive to the voice of God.

It was in January 2008 when I ewent through one of the most vulnerable and broken seasons of my life. At that time, a riot had broken out in the prison I was being housed at. One group of inmates assaulted another group, which in turn led to a prison riot. The US National Guard was called in, locking down the entire prison for forty days.

Anytime a prison is on lockdown, no one from the outside can come in, and no one on the inside can leave. Telephones and TVs are shut down, cutting off all contact with the free world. During this time, I could only write my girlfriend, but she never wrote back. I was miserable for those forty days.

Finally, when the lockdown was over and I was able to call home, I was excited because I thought my girlfriend would be happy to hear from me. But to my surprise, after a minute of conversation, I sensed that she either didn't want to talk to me or was with someone and couldn't talk freely. In the middle of our conversation, the phone went dead. She had hung up on me.

The rule was that inmates had to wait 30 minutes between phone calls. So, I waited and called her back, but she wouldn't answer the phone. I knew something wasn't right. I continued calling her repeatedly, but she still refused to answer.

The next day, I called again. A guy answered her phone. As soon as I recognized a man's voice, I growled, "Who is this?"

"Don't worry about who it is. She doesn't want to talk, but you won't stop calling."

I slammed down the phone. In disbelief and despair, I ran back to my bed, got under the covers, and cried. Then and there I declared war to sever the soul tie. As I remained crying under the covers, I prayed, "God . . . I'm done! If you'll just give me the strength, I will never call her again. She's gotten me out of her, and I'm ready to get her out of me!"

Seconds later, I heard a voice in my mind: *"I'll help you if you agree not to contact her for the rest of the time that you're in prison. No interruptions, no interactions, no distractions, and no interfer-*

ences. I don't want you to talk to another woman for the rest of the time that you're in prison."

I agreed. That's when God started giving me the blueprint on how to sever the soul tie.

Sever means "1) to divide by cutting or slicing, especially suddenly or forcibly; 2) to put an end to a connection or relationship, to break off; and 3) to become separated, divide or keep apart."[3] When severing a soul tie, you must know and understand that the person from whom you are disconnecting doesn't have the right or the power to remain in your life until they are ready to leave. You have to know, the ball is in your court. Therefore, you must initiate the severing if you're going to get free.

If you've ever been in a toxic and unfruitful relationship that constantly took you on an emotional roller-coaster ride, then what made you think the person would simply walk out of your life after you two created a pattern of dysfunction throughout the entire relationship? You are the one who must kill your fear, be bold, and eliminate every opportunity for that person to walk back into your life anytime they want to.

In other words, you must block their number and "unfollow" them from any social-media platforms. You must throw away the clothes they left at your house, burn the photos of you two together, erase all the messages and memories of them from your phone, eliminate the fragrances that remind you of them, stop going to their favorite restaurants, and refuse to listen to any songs that helped you create memories with them. When you truly declare war, your mindset should be, *"I must kill everything pertaining to them, because if I don't, then they will continue to kill me."* The longer you let anything that pertains to this person live, the longer you will stay connected to them mentally and emotionally.

It's crazy how a song can take you back to the memories of great times. It's crazy how a happy picture can cause you to forget about the hurt, pain, and betrayal they caused you. It's intoxicating to know that a scent they used to wear can cause you to want to call them and invite them over for coffee.

One of the laws of nature says that whatever you feed will live, but whatever you starve will die. At this point, you can't give yourself any excuse not to cut off (starve) every shape, form, or way of communication. I understand you may have kids together, but I'm sure you can work something out with the grandparents, family members, and mutual friends that will allow you to deal with the shared parenting issues. If you have the will, you will find a way.

You've been given instructions to guard your heart. By any means necessary, refuse them access to reconnect to you once you've decided to eradicate them from your life. Anytime you're serious about severing a soul tie, you must make this statement with absolute conviction: *"Fasting or detoxing myself from this ungodly soul tie is not an option; it's an absolute Commandment!"* If you give them the option to run in and out of your life, then every time you allow yourself to reconnect, and they hurt you again, the heartbreak is going to feel even worse. Plus, it will get even harder to re-sever the soul tie.

When you allow yourself to reconnect with this person before you've totally severed the soul tie, it's like breaking your fast or detox before it's complete. You were disobedient and didn't follow instructions fully; therefore, the effects of your disobedience will only make your consequences worse. Don't forget that you can't receive some blessings from God unless you finish what you started.

You will not get them out of you until you're fully detoxed; a partial detox doesn't work. During your detox or fast from the soul tie, the one thing it will show you is that the longer you remain disconnected from them physically, mentally, and emotionally, you are reclaiming the power you lost during the relationship. One of the worst feelings in the world is knowing in your head that you have power but not having the heart to use it. So instead of wielding your power to disconnect, you let the fear of losing them cause you to accept their abuse.

For every single day that you fast or detox from a relationship, you'll see that you are a lot stronger than you gave yourself credit for. The most powerful element of fasting and detoxing from an ungodly soul tie is operating in the divine exchange. For most people, during this time, their focus is disconnecting and getting the person out of them emotionally and mentally, but the greatest and most powerful part is what you fill yourself with as you dismiss this person and your relationship. In other words, you never displace without replacing. You're not subtracting but substituting.

THE AGENDA: CHANGE YOUR PERSPECTIVE

While you do the work to get the other person out of you, you must see them from the right perspective. In other words, you must see them for who they really are. If you don't change your perspective to gain a correct view of them, then you will keep them on a pedestal. Many people cannot disconnect and separate themselves from an ungodly soul tie or a dysfunctional relationship because they continue to see their mates as their "king" or "queen." Even though they may be separated or divorced physically, one person may still perceive the other as their "spouse" or "best friend."

Regarding spiritual warfare and severing soul ties, God can't deliver you from your friends; He will only deliver you from your enemies. You tell your friends, not your enemies, your secrets. You tell your friends, not your enemies, your plans. You tell your friends, not your enemies, your vision and mission. Therefore, until you can see the person as the enemy, God will never deliver you from them. If that sounds a bit harsh, let me remind you that you declared war against the ungodly soul tie, and war is harsh.

Anytime you declare war, you must see the other person as an enemy. We've been taught to express love to others, but the truth is there is a time to express your hatred for something (Ecclesiastes 3:8). I'm not telling you to hate this person, but I am telling you to hate the *spirit* that the person partnered with, which is causing the hurt and pain in your life. They may be a good person, but they weren't a good person to you, which is why you're severing the soul tie and getting them out of you.

The longer you meditate on how good they were to you, and all the good times you shared, the more you'll continue to see their potential. Then you'll hang onto a loving perspective of them, secretly hoping that they will change and become what you see in them.

Some people are married to the potential picture of their mates but do not see the reality of them. While it's great to see a person's potential, you must consider the reality of the person with whom you are living. Therefore, if you're going to sever a soul tie, then you must see them as they are and as who they've been to you. If you are divorced, then they are no longer your spouse. If you still see this person as your spouse, then you are telling yourself a lie, which will keep you tied. I know it's hard —especially if you were married for several years—but if you're going to break free, then you must face what you fear.

Why would you continue to torture yourself emotionally and mentally when they are gone and participating in physical, mental, financial, and emotional life with someone else? You are the only one who can take them off the pedestal you set them on in your mind. Before you can experience the power of your choice manifesting and happening in your life, you must decide in your heart.

After you change the way you see them, you must change the way you see yourself. You're not a victim; you're a victor! You're not a failure; you're more than a conqueror, and you're a winner. You're not weak; you're strong. You're not depressed; you're going through a process. The lie most people tell themselves goes something like this: *"I'm experiencing depression; therefore, I'm a depressed person. My marriage failed; therefore, I'm a failure. I feel like a victim in this situation; therefore, I must be a victim."*

These are lies. What you are going through doesn't have anything to do with who God says you are. Your identity doesn't come from the storms, trials, tribulations, or tests you experience. Your identity comes from voice of God and Word of God. If you don't see yourself the way God sees you, that ungodly soul tie will take advantage of you.

I once counseled a young man by the name of Chris. Chris took me out to breakfast one morning because he wanted advice on whether he should ask his girlfriend to marry him or let the relationship go. As the conversation began, he said that they had been together for four years, but for the last two years, their relationship had been on the rocks.

He allowed her to move into his condo after eight months of dating because they both wanted to save money. They agreed to split the bills in half and go half on all the groceries. After four months, she got laid off from her job, and it took three months before she found employment again. While she was unemployed, Chris paid all the bills, including her car loan.

To his surprise, when she started her new job, she told Chris that if they were planning to get married in the future, then he should manage all the bills, as if they were already married. Chris agreed.

About six months later, problems arose. One day his girlfriend was in the shower and her phone rang. It was on the counter next to Chris, so he was able to see the caller's name on the screen: Harold. This piqued his curiosity, so decided to check her messages. To his surprise, she had changed her password.

His suspicion skyrocketed. He didn't say anything to her right then. Instead, he put on his detective hat. He bought a phone and put it in the trunk of her car, using it as a tracking device. A week later, she said that she was going out to have drinks with her girlfriends. Chris followed her via the tracking phone in her trunk.

She drove to a restaurant that was forty-five minutes on the other side of town. Chris watched her as she had dinner with a man. When they left the restaurant, Chris watched the man walk her to the car. As soon as they embraced and kissed, he started his car and quickly pulled up in front of them. Chris jumped out of the car and went after the guy while his girlfriend stood in shock. By the grace of God, Chris didn't go to jail.

As crazy as it may sound, he allowed his girlfriend to continue living in his apartment while Chris kept paying all the bills.

Over the past couple of years, Chis had caught his girlfriend with Harold again. Chris has forgiven her because he loves her and wants to work things out with her. He told her that they would have to get into a church, go to counseling, and leave the past behind—including Harold. They stopped by our church to visit one Sunday, but they came only one time and refused to come back.

As Chris told me his story, I sensed that he was a great guy who had connected with the wrong girl.

"What should I do, Pastor James?"

I was 100% honest with him. "Chris, when you started the conversation, you had me thinking that you needed to know if you should marry her because you were convicted about your shacking up with her, but in all actuality, you're trying to marry her because you think that after marriage, she'll stop cheating on you. If you want to know my opinion, then I'll give it to you."

"Please, Pastor, tell me the truth. I value your opinion," Chris said.

"You don't need to marry her because she doesn't respect you. She doesn't love you, and it sounds to me like she won't accept your ring or invitation to marry her. You need to let her go and start a brand-new life."

"You don't think that she can grow to respect and love me?"

"Yes, she can, but she doesn't see you as a man worthy of respect and honor right now," I said.

"Pastor, how do I walk away after four years of giving my life to her?"

"Look at it this way, Chris. You haven't lost anything, but you have learned a lot of things. Hear me and hear me well. If you don't see yourself the way God sees you, your girlfriend, or anyone else, will continue to take advantage of you and use you until you have nothing left of yourself."

Chris studied me for a moment. "Pastor, you're right. It seems that all she's done is take from me since day one. What do I need to do to move on?"

"Once you've decided to move on, you're going to have to get pregnant with a vision for your future that's 100% bigger than your past."

THE WEAPON: YOUR GOD-GIVEN VISION

It's vital that you see the ungodly soul tie as the enemy as well as see yourself the way God sees you. Become pregnant with a God-given vision. The Bible says, *"Where there is no vision, the people perish"* (Proverbs 29:18). If you don't have a vision ahead of you that's greater than everything behind you, you'll be tempted to look back and return to what was familiar.

When God wants to bring you out of an ungodly relationship or an ungodly soul tie, then He will give you a mental picture of your future, so you don't remain in bondage to the person or soul tie. Once I chose a journey of transformation, God showed me a vision of the direction in which He wanted my life to flow, and who He wanted me to become. Even though God gave me a vision, it was still my choice to accept it, partner with God, and walk out of the picture that I was seeing.

At first, I didn't know just how powerful the vision was. But as soon as I started following the vision, it started changing me into another man. The vision I saw on the inside changed my reading material on the outside. The vision I saw on the inside changed my conversations on the outside. The vision I saw on the inside changed the TV shows I watched on the outside. The vision I saw on the inside changed the kinds of friendships I had on the outside. The vision I saw on the inside changed how I saw myself as a person. The vision I saw on the inside made me walk in confidence on the outside.

Whenever people receive a conviction of their God-given vision, following that vision will govern, control, direct, and change every dimension of their lives. Vision is the tool that God uses so we won't have an empty or idle mind. Vision will replace the person you are displacing out of your life.

When a vision becomes your obsession, that's when you will be on the pathway to transformation. A God-given vision is designed to pull you out of who used to be and turn you into who God is calling you to be. If you ever become one with the God-given vision, expect your attitude to shift, and your altitude in life to accelerate. Your vision will not eliminate all pain, but that vision will keep you focused until you outgrow the pain.

Filling up with God's vision for your future will separate you from ungodly confusion. In other words, the weapon you need to sever the ungodly soul ties is a godly self-perception and a new vision for the future. If you can see something new, you can become someone new, and you can leave behind and eliminate anything or anyone who is part of your old life.

CHAPTER 14

LIES THAT KEEP YOU TIED

WHAT IF I told you that the secret of your ungodly soul tie is rooted in a lie? It's worth repeating that lies are a major weapon Satan uses against the body of Christ. As Jesus was speaking to the Jews, he said, *"For you are the children of your father the devil, and you love to do the evil things he does. He was a murderer from the beginning. He has always hated the truth because there is no truth in him. When he lies, it is consistent with his character, for he is a liar and the father of lies"* (John 8:44 [NLT]).

Jesus said that Satan is a liar and the father of lies. This tells me that the kingdom of darkness is built on lies. Jesus told his disciples, *"I am the Way, the Truth, and the Life. No one can come to the Father except through Me"* (John 14:6 [NLT]). Notice that Jesus calls himself "the Truth." Since Jesus identifies himself as Truth, the kingdom of light must be built on truth.

Listen to what Jesus said to his disciples: *"And I will pray to the Father, and He will give you another helper, that He may abide with you forever: the Spirit of Truth, whom the world cannot receive because it neither sees Him nor knows Him, but you know Him, for He dwells with you and will be in you"* (John 14:16-17 [NKJV]).

In this scripture, Jesus calls Holy Spirit "the Spirit of truth." Also, Jesus said to the Jews who believed in him, *"If ye continue in My Word, then are ye My disciples indeed, and ye shall know the truth, and the truth shall make you free"* (John 8:31-32). The first word Jesus uses here is the word "if." "If" is found 1522 times in the Bible, and all of them express a condition. Jesus was telling these new Jewish believers (and us), *"If* you're going to remain as true disciples and have freedom from sin, [*then*] you must continue in my word." If they were to continue in his Word, they would eventually make it to the next level of truth.

This means that if they refused to continue in His Word, then they would have remained in bondage to a lie. Jesus went on to say, *"And ye shall know the truth, and the truth shall make you free."* Here's the point: Truth leads to freedom, and lies lead to bondage. For most people, the quickest and greatest deliverance that will set them free from an ungodly soul tie is the truth.

In contrast, a lie keeps you bound, attached, and tied to an ungodly soul tie. As soon as you accept the truth, the lie must die in your heart and soul. The biggest enemy of an ungodly soul tie is the truth.

As I've continued in His Word, I've discovered 10 lies that keep us bound to an ungodly soul tie. Let's expose them so that you will know the truth and no longer be bound by lies.

LIE #1: ONE DAY, THEY WILL SEE THAT I AM THE BEST THING THAT EVER HAPPENED TO THEM.

Often, when one's heart has been broken by a mate or spouse, and they refuse to let go of the marriage or relationship, they will tell themselves things to feel better about keeping hope alive. They're not ready to fully let go of that person or that relationship—even though it is dead and unfruitful, or their mate or spouse walked away a long time ago.

To be honest, you may be right when you told yourself that you were the best thing to ever happen to them, but you must ask yourself, *"What if my mate's eyes never open to see that I was the best thing to ever happen to them? What if they don't care that I was the best thing that ever happened to them? What if they don't think I was the best thing to ever happen to them? What if they believe that they will find someone who will be better to them than I was?"*

If your mate is thinking along the lines of any of these questions, then you are telling yourself a lie. Therefore, you will remain tied. It's dangerous, delusional, and destructive to try to think for someone else when you're wrestling with brokenness or defeat within yourself. If you're not strong enough to face the truth, you'll remain in bondage to a lie. You must face the fact that what you had together is over, and there will not be a resurrection of this marriage or relationship.

Also, you're living in deceit anytime you try to assume the thoughts of someone who's not trying to reconnect with you. While trying to assume their thoughts from a place of hurt, you're trapping yourself in a delusional mindset.

LIE #2: THEY'RE STILL MY SPOUSE

I've counseled multiple individuals who were married for several years before separating or divorcing. I've also counseled people who've been in a relationship for 20+ years but were never married.

Ironically, during our conversations, many would say things like, "I know we are not together, but I still see him as my husband," or "I know we broke up and are no longer together, but in my heart, she's still my wife." Every time I hear these or similar statements, it's hard for me to look that person in the eyes and tell them, "The divorce is final, and as hard as it is to accept, the truth is that they are not your spouse."

In these delicate situations, if I speak the truth but don't speak it in love, then the situation will become even more fatal. If I console a person with a lot of love but do not speak the truth, then I am ushering them into a deeper level of failure. My prayer is that if you're in this situation, then I hope you can feel the Love of God flowing from these words as I give you this truth. I know it's hard to receive, but God loves you more than any human being could ever love you. Nevertheless, He will not withhold His truth from you because it's the tool He uses to heal you and make you whole.

Maybe you're wondering if God can change your former spouse's mind. Absolutely! God can do anything, but the real question is, will God go against his Word and interfere with the person's free will? If God goes against that person's free will, He violates His Word. If God violates His Word, it makes Him a liar. And only two things God can't do: He can't lie, and He can't fail.

If you have made up your mind that you want the unhealthy soul tie completely out of your soul, my challenge to you in love is to accept the truth that your spouse's time is up in your life. You don't deserve continual verbal, mental, physical, or financial abuse.

About seven months before I was to be released from federal prison, I was still making excuses for why my ex-girlfriend had left me for another man. Because I was telling one of my good friends how I wasn't going to rekindle the relationship with her when I got released, he made me accept the truth so I could destroy the lie and untangle the ungodly soul tie.

One day we were talking about why I felt like she had left me. I blamed her leaving me on four things: (1) I went to prison; (2) I couldn't continue to take care of her; (3) I had cheated on her in the past, and (4) She didn't like my mom.

My friend stopped me and said, "Bruh, you're on your way home, and you've changed your life. I cannot let you leave this prison, so you can go back to that girl and fall flat on your face. Stop lying to yourself, bro. She didn't leave you because you cheated on her in the past; she didn't leave you because you couldn't take care of her anymore; she didn't leave you because you got locked up or because she doesn't get along with your mom. Let's be real. She left you because she doesn't want you anymore! She left you because your time in her life was up, and she left you because that's what she wanted to do—leave you! I wouldn't be your true friend if I allowed you to keep believing these lies. Come on, bro, face it! This is for your freedom and your future. Until you face the truth, you're going to go back out there and breathe life into that lie. Please, let the lie die, so God can give you the strength to start a new life."

As hard as it was to receive the truth, it was exactly what I had to accept. Instantaneously, I felt a weight drop off my chest when I said, "Jim, you're right! She doesn't want me anymore, and my time is up in her life."

LIE #3: YOU CAN'T HELP WHOM YOU FALL IN LOVE WITH.

Usually, when people say this to themselves or others, they feel powerless and stuck in the pain. They want to make progress faster than they are making it, but since it doesn't feel like they are getting free, they give an excuse to go back and try to rekindle with their ex.

The truth is that you can control who you fall in love with. Before you fell in love, you chose to accept what you were feeling and believed that this person would fulfill every promise and covenant they made to you. In other words, love is a choice. Separation is a choice. Divorce is a choice. And removing their soul out of you is a choice.

Would you like to know the sequence of the soul (i.e., how the soul operates)? You hear a word, thought, advice, or see a picture. Whether it's right or wrong, you think about it and develop your interpretation. From there, you accept your interpretation. Next, you believe it. Then you feel it, which turns into a conviction. A conviction leads to a philosophy. You make decisions based on your philosophy. Your decision turns into action. Continual action develops a habit. Habits become your lifestyle. Your lifestyle determines your character. In the end, your character leads you to your destiny.

In the beginning, you accepted that your emotions were getting attached to this person, but you never challenged what you were accepting and believing. Now that this person is gone, you can reject those unhealthy emotions that are trying to remain alive within you. Yes, you can stop, stall, and stagnate those old emotions! The more you keep feeding yourself a new mindset, the more your new vision and life will grow. That love is old; now, God is giving you something brand-new! It may take some time but this will work if you work it.

LIE #4: THEY LOVE THEIR FAMILY TOO MUCH NOT TO COME BACK TO US.

When kids are involved, you would think that breakups, separations, and divorces seem impossible. This is true also with ties to parents or in-laws. The fact is that it's not easy to let go. What's scary about this is that just because you will sacrifice and stay for the sake of the family, that doesn't necessarily mean that they will sacrifice and stay for the sake of the family, too. You can't make assumptions based on what you would do in a situation because they are not you. What if they're not who you think they are? What if their values have changed? What if their goal or perspective has changed to something unhealthy? Should they come back for the kids' sake? Maybe, but will they? The answer remains a mystery.

I've been both the victim and the assailant in an ungodly soul tie. When you're the assailant, usually selfishness and self-centeredness are your priority. Nothing or no one else matters more than getting what you want, when you want it, and how you want it. Usually, sin, greed, arrogance, and pride are the driving forces of this attitude.

You can know the problem that they are dealing with, but that doesn't mean you can change it. Your job isn't to focus on why they don't love the family enough to sacrifice and come back home; your assignment is to let it go, so you can outgrow the pain, hurt, and betrayal and be a better parent to your children, as well as a better person for yourself.

When you assume that one day, they'll come back to you because of the kids or the family, you are accepting that you will still be second place in their life. Anytime you're not in first place in the physical realm—because God is in first place in the spiritual realm—the relationship or the marriage is dysfunctional. If you're married, then it's the order of God for you to be in first place to your spouse, not your kids, because one day, your kids will become adults and leave your home. Therefore, if your spouse or mate can't put you first, then you'll never be #1 in their life. If you can't be in first place, then it's time to look forward to who you will be in first place with in your new life.

LIE #5: I CANNOT LIVE WITHOUT THEM

This one is dangerous because when you tell yourself that you can't live without someone, you've subconsciously slipped into idolatry; that is, the relationship, marriage, or other person has become your god. If this person has become your god, then they have become an enemy to God in your life. Anything or anyone who takes priority over God the Father in your life has become an idol. In both the Old and New Testaments, the First and greatest Commandment is to have no other gods (Exodus 20:3) and to love God with all your heart, soul, and mind (Matthew 22:37).

These scriptures inform us that God will not allow anything or any person to take first place in our hearts. Believing that you can't live without that other person is giving yourself over to that person, and you've become their servant.

Believing this lie is one reason people stay in unfruitful, ungodly, and dysfunctional relationships for decades. It is also why many people tolerate continual adultery, verbal and physical abuse, and addictions from their mates. People who believe this lie accept the worst of their mate's behavior. Then they will allow this unfruitful behavior to turn them into a dysfunctional and unfruitful person.

Let me pause here and issue a caution: Please don't get selective hearing or think that I am an advocate for divorce. This book is for people who aren't married but are tied to an ungodly soul tie and have decided to get free. This book is also for people going through a divorce, who want to get the spouse out of them, so they can start their new lives. This book is also for those who are single physically but living with their former mate mentally and emotionally. Whatever category you are in, you're sick and tired of this person living within you, so your main pursuit is to get rid of them internally.

Remember, if you don't uncover the lie and accept the truth, then you'll continue to remain tied. God created us for relationships¾*healthy* relationships¾but God didn't create us to be dependent on others; rather, He created us to be dependent on Him. Therefore, it's time to stop telling yourself that you can't live without the other person. Remember, the God of the Universe lives inside you, so you are never alone.

LIE #6: IT WASN'T SUPPOSED TO END LIKE THIS.

This lie is powerful because it is tied to the vision you had for your life. You saw yourself growing old with the other person. You saw yourself building something together that is greater than the two of you separately, and for a while, it looked like that was happening. You saw yourself having huge family gatherings with them for the rest of your life. You saw yourself creating and leaving a legacy with them.

Now that what you saw is shattered, you keep thinking, *"It wasn't supposed to end like this."* The question you must ask yourself is, *"How long will I continue to hold onto my vision now that I know it was not theirs?"* Maybe it used to be their vision, but today it isn't, because they're gone and not coming back. Therefore, it's regressive if you continue to think about what was or could've been. In contrast, it's progressive to think about the possibilities of what can be with someone new. What happened to you is behind you, but what and whom God has for you is ahead of you. You cannot reach what's in your future while holding onto what's in your past.

Therefore, vision is vital and brings victory. You will eliminate the memories by filling yourself with the imagination of what could be. You will find life, strength, excitement, joy, and new expectations in your vision of the future. God gives you the ability to operate in the preview (i.e., imagination), so you don't have to remain in bondage to the replay (i.e., old, unfruitful memories).

I encourage you to meditate on Jeremiah 29:11: *"'For I know the plans I have for you,' says the Lord. 'They are plans for good, and not for disaster, to give you a future and a hope'"* (NLT). God knew this day was coming in your life because He is omniscient (all-knowing) and omnipotent (all-power). Therefore, since He's all-knowing and all-power, don't you think He wants to see His child (you) healed, blessed, and made whole? Yes! He abso-lutely does!

So, God is thinking things about you that you're not thinking about yourself. Therefore, all you must do is eliminate the lie that "it wasn't supposed to end like this."

Next, ask God, "Father, would you please tell me just one thing that You are thinking about me?" Make a deal with God and tell Him that if He tells you one of his thoughts about you, then you'll release the thought that's not adding value to your life.

Come on, soldier! You've declared war! Now, it's time to get rid of this lie! It's a lie because the relationship *did* end "like this." It's a lie because you cannot control this other person. Therefore, the only way that the thought, "It wasn't supposed to end like this," could be true is if they agreed with you throughout the entirety of the journey. Accept that they didn't agree that "it wasn't supposed to end like this." As soon as you accept this truth, the lie will die.

LIE #7: GOD WILL NEVER FORGIVE ME FOR THIS DIVORCE.

This lie is a big one that the enemy uses to make a child of God feel unworthy, unacceptable, and unforgiven. It's a lie that the spirit of religion uses against the Body of Christ. God hates divorce (Malachi 2:6 [NKJV]), but God also has a deep and unconditional love for His children (John 3:16; 1 John 3:1). Though God hates divorce, He still loves the people who are unfortunate enough to go through a divorce.

According to Jesus, *"All sins shall be forgiven unto the sons of men, and blasphemers wherewith soever they shall blaspheme"* (Mark 3:28). I believe that the Body of Christ has made people feel that if they get a divorce, God will not forgive them, and some people have been led to believe that God hates them, and they are going to hell because they have gotten a divorce.

Please, don't think this is your license to divorce. This is a truth God wants his children to know so they can walk in freedom and not bondage. Romans 8:1 says, *"There is therefore now no condemnation to them which are in Christ Jesus."* If you are in Christ, he doesn't condemn you.

You cannot control that your spouse has committed and continues to commit adultery against you. You cannot control that your spouse continues to neglect, abuse, and abandon you. You simply cannot control that your spouse doesn't want to remain married to you. Just because you're divorced, or you're going through a divorce, doesn't mean that God has not and will not forgive you. Jesus said, *"The thief cometh not but for to steal, kill, and destroy; I have come that they might have life, and that they might have it more abundantly"* (John 10:10). This life He's talking about also refers to emotional and personal wholeness.

It's not the Will of God for us to live in depression, defeat, and despair because of other people's adultery, abuse, neglect, or unhealthy addictions. God is a God of fruitfulness. Every marriage has its struggles, bruises, bumps, or challenges, but the purpose of marriage is for both people to be fruitful. If a person leaves you, then you can't make them come back to you.

If your spouse has divorced or is divorcing you, it doesn't mean that God is divorcing you or that God will not forgive you. He hates divorce, but He still loves divorcees. Therefore, God will always forgive His child who comes back to Him and chooses His ways, despite the sin or the mistake. Accept the truth that God loves you first for who you are, not because of what you do.

LIE #8: WE'RE JUST TAKING A BREAK; EVENTUALLY, WE WILL GET BACK TOGETHER.

If you are telling yourself this, then ask yourself, "Am I ready to close the door and sever this ungodly soul tie?" It sounds like to me you're keeping hope alive. If so, then answer this: "How long am I going to keep the door cracked open?"

Let me remind you that keeping the door cracked open allows options for an ungodly soul tie. If they can call or see you whenever they want to, then it won't be long before you allow them back into your bed whenever they want to be. Maybe you're also telling yourself, "It wasn't the right time when we got together, but we will get back together in the future." Maybe you're right. However, you must also consider how many other soul ties they may have created or are currently creating before they come back to you. If you believe that they'll come back better, then you must also accept that they may instead come back worse.

While you're taking a break, are you growing in the same direction or growing apart? If you're exploring the possibilities of the good, please don't neglect the possibilities of the bad. To the person who's declared war on the ungodly soul tie while believing this lie, you're double-minded, uncertain, and indecisive. Therefore, you're still tied. God cannot do any work until you make up your mind to be done with being tied to an ungodly soul tie.

LIE #9: ALL RELATIONSHIPS ARE DYSFUNCTIONAL; THERE IS NO SUCH THING AS A PERFECT RELATIONSHIP.

You may be right, but you're wrestling with double-mindedness , comparison, and silent competition. Just because you think all relationships are dysfunctional doesn't mean they always are. If you grew up around or in dysfunctional relationships, then you might believe that having a peaceful and prosperous relationship is impossible.

Sometimes we've been so conditioned by the counterfeit for so long that when the truth comes, we think it's a lie. Dysfunction has shaped our lives to such a degree that peace is wrong; it could scare us. A relationship doesn't have to be constant disagreements, arguments, fighting, or frequent breakups. Because some people are accustomed to that type of ongoing dysfunction, when their mate says, "I'm done!" it's hard for them to believe.

If you're waiting for your mate to come back into the dysfunctional relationship while they have no intention of doing so, you might feel lonely and unworthy. Don't be surprised if you think that you'll never find true love. Dysfunction breeds dysfunction. Chaos breeds chaos, and lies breed liars.

The only way for you to find true love is to cross over from a chaotic world into a peaceful world. If you don't, then you'll never find what you truly desire. Maybe it's a blessing that you separated from this ungodly soul tie. Maybe God saved you from a life of drama, hurt, pain, and brokenness. If this resonates with you, then I believe you've been given a personal invitation to enter a season of isolation, so you can do internal cleaning and healing.

I hope you are tired of being in chaotic relationships and are ready to experience and embrace a new type of love. It's a love that's honest, respectful, peaceful, joyful, full of new exposure, and filled with blessings. To receive this, refuse what you are used to, change the way you think, and choose—it's time to date up!

You can't continue to do life in a dysfunctional relationship. Attempt to do life in the place you want to be. It may at first feel uncomfortable and sometimes unattainable, but you can be it only if you can see it. You don't have to live by the negative things you see on the outside. If you can be exposed to a new reality on the inside, it will become your reality on the outside.

The truth is, every relationship is not dysfunctional, but you will continue to believe that lie if you don't get a new world to see.

LIE #10: EVENTUALLY, THEY WILL LEAVE THEIR MATE FOR ME.

If you are the third party to a marriage ("the side chick or her sugar daddy") , and you've gotten tied emotionally, mentally, and sexually, then you may believe they will leave their current spouse for you.

I had a friend whose aunt dated a married man and had children with him. Their affair went on for 20+ years. She went to her grave thinking that one day, he would leave his wife and marry her.

If your ungodly soul tie were to leave their spouse and marry you, then life would make sure that you would not have any peace, joy, happiness, or pure, divine love. If you start a relationship in adultery, then eventually it will end in destruction.

Whatsoever a person sows, that is exactly what that person will reap.

They're not your spouse. It's time to repent and ask God for forgiveness so you can start a new life. You shouldn't want anyone who isn't yours. You are smarter than that. You are wiser than that. You are more beautiful than that, and you are more loved than that. If you're stuck in that lie, you're not in divine love but trapped in perverted lust. My purpose is to tell you that God wants to heal every broken place in you. Plus, He wants to make you whole. If you fit this description, Holy Spirit is speaking directly to you.

God wants you to know that He hates the sin, but He still loves you. He will receive you, love you, and heal you. One of the most powerful things you have as a believer in Jesus is your belief system. Jesus said, *"All things are possible to him that believeth"* (Mark 9:23). Your beliefs will either keep you bound to this ungodly soul tie or kill and dismantle this ungodly soul tie. The choice is yours.

Maybe you're believing a lie that I haven't mentioned. Whatever the lie, it's keeping you tied.

Now is the time to admit the lie and accept the truth, so the lie will die. If you keep believing the lie, then your soul will remain tied to what's unhealthy and ungodly. However, if you receive the truth, then freedom is the first fruit that you will produce. All you need to do is find the lie, untangle it, and develop a new truth. From there, I promise you'll lighten the load of this ungodly soul tie or sever it completely.

CHAPTER 15

THE FIGHT TO FORGIVE

THE HARDEST BRIDGE TO cross in the most intense battle of your war to sever unhealthy or ungodly soul ties is getting rid of that toxic, wasteful, harmful, and infectious disease called unforgiveness. It's a nonnegotiable to destroy unforgiveness. When you do, you experience healing and wholeness throughout your being. Therefore, the enemy and your flesh will fight you with every weapon in its arsenal to keep you in unforgiveness.

Remember, to win the war of severing the soul tie, you must have an agenda, a strategy, and the necessary weapons to defeat the enemy. It may surprise you to learn that the most powerful weapon in your arsenal is the choice to forgive the person or people you are/were tied to.

Usually, after you've been hurt, bruised, battered, or betrayed by a person whom you've become one with, instead of forgiving that person, it's human nature to blame them for the pain you're experiencing, but the byproduct of blaming someone else for your pain will produce envy, bitterness, resentment, rage, and hatred. All these negative elements are the fruit of unforgiveness, and they keep you stuck, unable to move toward your God-given destiny.

I learned the hard way that unforgiveness is a heart issue and a representation of a negative pride problem. This heart issue will stop, stagnate, and stall your ability to sever the soul tie. Forgiveness is a choice, and the longer you refuse to forgive, the longer you will remain tied. Jesus said to his disciples:

> "It is impossible, but that offences will come, but woe unto him through whom they come! It were better for him that a millstone were hanged about his neck, and he cast into the sea, than that he should offend one of these little ones. Take heed to yourselves: If thy brother trespass against thee, rebuke him, and if he repents, forgive him, and if he trespasses against thee seven times in a day, and seven times in a day turns again to thee, saying, 'I repent,' thou shalt forgive him. And the apostles said unto the Lord, 'Increase our faith.'"
>
> — LUKE 17:1-5

In Luke 17:1, Jesus said, *"It is impossible, but that offenses will come."* He means that in life, there is no way of avoiding someone offending you. Everyone will be offended by someone. Your parents, kids, friends, spouse, mate, coworkers, or even a stranger will offend you one day. The definition of *offense* is "to cause a person or people to feel hurt, angry or upset by something they said or did to you."[1]

Therefore, it's easy to be offended by your spouse or mate if they betrayed, abandoned, neglected, or rejected you. Jesus alerts us to be prepared for such an offense; therefore, He expects us to forgive them. This is why Jesus said in Luke 17:4, *"And if he trespasses against thee seven times in a day, and seven times in a day turns again to thee, saying, 'I repent,' thou shalt forgive him."* Jesus is not focused on the number of times that you should forgive a person, but that children of God are people of forgiveness. Forgiveness is not a one-time event but a lifestyle and a mindset. God has forgiven us for every past, present, and future sin (Psalms 103:12; 1 John 1:9; 1 John 2:2), and He expects us to forgive others (Matthew 6:14). Your act of forgiveness can work to destroy the enemy, or it can work to destroy you.

The word "forgive" means "(1) a deliberate decision to let go of the offense and vengeance towards someone who has hurt, harmed, or betrayed you; (2) a conscious choice to cancel the debt; and (3) the decision to eliminate every expectation that you had for the person who hurt you."

The first definition of forgiveness tells us that we must let go. Let go of the betrayal, rejection, abandonment, abuse, and neglect. That's hard to do if we are entertaining conversations, discussions, and movies that remind you of what a person did to you.

One day my wife, Tiffaney, gave a powerful revelation about offense and forgiveness, which, if you accept it, will accelerate your healing process. One Sunday during our morning worship service, she said, "It's dangerous to listen to truth—when you're hearing it and your spirit is crushed." We had gone through a hurtful situation. My wife was angry, and her spirit was deeply crushed by what the person had done. Therefore, she got on YouTube and started listening to messages about betrayal, vindication, God making her enemies her footstool, and how God was going to prepare a table before her in the presence of her enemies. She was listening to truth, but her spirit was crushed.

Consequently, the truth she was hearing drove her to pray against her enemies rather than praying for her enemies. She was hearing truth, but perverting it because her spirit was crushed. As she was listening to truth from the place of hurt, the Holy Spirit spoke to her: *Do you think that I care more about vindication than I care about reconciliation? You're praying for my wrath to touch them, but you need to be praying for my love to touch them.*

You will remain broken, crushed, and confused when you listen to a truth that empowers brokenness. You will fail to know how to let the offense go. It's not wise to try to figure out how God will defend you, but it's a demonstration of the love of God when you pray for God to save your enemies.

Therefore, even though you hear the truth and want God to vindicate you, be wise and listen to messages about love and letting go of offenses. Now may not be the season for you to listen to the truth as it pertains to vindication because you may not know how to filter it through a lens of love. You can't control what others did to you in the past, but you can control what you receive into your heart now and in the future.

Letting go may not be easy, but I guarantee you, it's worth it. Continuing to carry the weight of unforgiveness, bitterness, resentment, envy, and hate is too heavy as you journey toward complete healing and wholeness. Let it go so you can grow.

The second definition of forgiveness is deliberately canceling the debt. You feel that your spouse owes you what they promised you. If you were married, then they owed you respect, honor, protection, provision, partnership, security, and love. If you weren't married to them, then you developed expectations without a covenant. Therefore, you took a greater risk of becoming one with a person without demanding that they enter a divine covenant with you. For the divorced person, your spouse did owe you these things. Unfortunately, now they don't owe you anything because it's a new day, and you cannot continue living according to an invalid covenant.

I'm not being insensitive, but my assignment is to bring you to a truth, which will open your eyes and make you free (if you accept it). What happened is in the past. You can't go back and redo it, but you can use the wisdom you learned to catapult yourself into the future.

I received a revelation about forty-five days away from being released from federal prison. God was preparing me to face one of the biggest obstacles to my personal freedom: my ex-girl-friend. On this day, I sat on my bed, wrestling with how I was going to remain strong and not get entangled back into the ungodly soul tie I had with her. I hadn't talked to her or seen her in over three and a half years. Unfortunately, I knew my soul was still attached to her. In my mind, I thought about all the materialistic things I had given her while I was in prison: money, jewelry, and a brand-new Cadillac Escalade EXT, which still had me attached to her. As I was thinking, a fleeting thought came across my mind: *Cancel the debt! She owes you nothing!*

My next thought was, *Oh yes, she owes me! Look at all the stuff I left her with. She's gotta pay me back.*

The voice came back and said, *The same way I canceled the debt of your sins, that I chose not to hold against you, I want you to cancel that materialistic debt you are holding against her. Let her go free.* That's when I knew it was the voice of God speaking to me.

Instantly I was shocked, not understanding, and almost paralyzed. I felt a deep conviction within. As I tried to keep reasoning, the voice spoke back to me one final time. *Holding that truck against her and feeling like she still owes you is the only thing you can use to stay connected to her. Let it go and cancel the debt.*

By then I was out of excuses. It was time for me to execute God's message to me.

About six months later, I was home from prison and sitting outside, having the final conversation with her.

I'll never forget when I looked her in the eyes and said, "You don't owe me anything!"

Immediately, it felt like I had cut off the enemy's head! Everything I thought I'd lost in that ungodly union had been restored to me in that moment. My confidence, identity, strength, boldness, self-love, self-acceptance, self-belief, and self-respect increased all at once. That's how I know one part of forgiveness is when you can honestly cancel the debt; not just saying casually, *"I forgive,"* but meaning it sincerely. When you truly mean it, every time you think about that person, you will say, *"They don't owe me anything."*

The third definition of forgiveness is "a decision to eliminate every expectation you have for the person who hurt, betrayed, rejected, or abandoned you." A person cannot move on and sever a soul tie if old expectations are still intact. This person is gone, but you still expect them to apologize to you. This person has started a new life with someone else, but you still expect them not to post about their love life on social media. They haven't talked to you in over a year, but you still expect them to call and check on you. They are living a new life, but you still expect them to be considerate of you.

You're still expecting certain things from them because you're still holding on to a fabricated reality of the past. If you've recognized this to be true, you must be telling yourself (and believe it), "How can I let go of these expectations when I don't know how to?" Honestly, you know how to let it go, but maybe you just don't want to.

However, if you don't know how to let go of old expectations, then start by asking yourself these questions:

- Should I expect something from this person when we are no longer together?
- Should I expect something from this person—even though I cannot control them?
- Should I expect something from this person when they don't believe they owe it to me? If this person knows they owe this to me, then will they ever give it to me?

If you answer no to any of these questions, then you've decided that the expectations you once had are not important enough to keep telling yourself a lie that has the power to keep you attached to them.

If you answer yes to any of these questions, then you're believing a lie, which is keeping you from moving forward into your God-designed future.

So, what do you do to squash these expectations? What does forgiveness look like?

For example, if you lended them money during the marriage or relationship, then let them have it. Don't expect them to pay you back. Forgive the debt. In this way, you will kill your expectations that they will return the money, and this will increase your ability to sever the tie.

Expectations keep you attached. What you do not destroy will eventually destroy you. What you do not master will eventually master you. What you do not conquer will eventually conquer you.

In other words, if you don't eliminate false expectations, eventually they will depress, defeat, and destroy every dimension of your life. Once again, accept the truth so that the lie will be forced to die.

If you pay attention to each definition of forgiveness, you will see the common denominator: decision, which informs us that forgiveness is not a feeling but a decision. Anytime I am in a coaching or counseling session and the call of action is forgiveness, most people say something like, "I forgave them, but for some reason, it doesn't feel like I have because every time I think about them, those feelings of anger and bitterness rise back up." That's when I explain in detail that forgiveness is not a feeling but a decision.

One day while I was on the phone with a close friend, Tom, who was struggling with forgiving our close mutual friend, Shawn, I had to break this down into simple yet powerful terms. Tom said, "James, I am struggling with this unforgiveness."

"Why do you think this is so?" I asked.

"Because today was the first day that I saw Shawn in a long time. I said I had forgiven him, but when I saw him, all that rage, bitterness, and hatred rose in me again. So, as soon as I caught myself, I said, *'I gotta call James and ask him if I forgave Shawn, then why do I still feel like I hate him?'"*

"That's a great question, Tom, but first, let me take you back to the scriptures. We must lay a solid foundation, and Jesus showed us in Mark 9:23 when He said, *'All things are possible to him that believeth.'* Understand that?"

"Yep, I got it," Tom said.

"So now my question to you is this: on the day that you decided to forgive Shawn, do you believe that deep down in your heart you did forgive him?"

"Absolutely! I forgave him," Tom said.

"But you just saw him for the first time in four months after you say you forgave him. Now those feelings of bitterness and unforgiveness are still rising up, right?"

"Yep, that's what happened," said Tom.

"How long did you harbor that unforgiveness and hate before you decided to forgive him?"

"Probably about two and a half years."

"Okay. So, now that you decided to forgive him, you expect the feelings of bitterness and unforgiveness to instantly disappear on the day that you forgave him? Bro, hear me! You don't have a forgiveness problem because you *did* forgive him. You're having a renewal-of-the-mind challenge, and a renewal-of-the-feelings challenge. Watch this, bro. If you truly decided to forgive him and did so, then that doesn't necessarily mean that the feelings of hatred and bitterness instantly left. If you continue to renew your mind to your decision to forgive, and if you continue to renew your mind to love him, and if you continue to renew your mind to let go of the offense, then the more you see him, and the more you continue to renew your mind, the more your thoughts and feelings will submit to your act of forgiveness.

"If you keep thinking about what he did to you, you're empowering the feelings of unforgiveness. On the other hand, just because you feel like you didn't forgive him doesn't mean that you didn't forgive him. The question is this, whose report will you believe? Will you believe that you truly forgave him? I'm not telling you that your feelings are not real, but I am saying that your feelings will lie to you; your feelings are not you, your decision, or your actions. Those feelings will challenge your decision and let you know that you haven't renewed your mind completely.

"This is what you need to do every time you see him and think about him: Reinforce your decision by opening your mouth and saying aloud, *'Shawn doesn't owe me anything. I have forgiven Shawn, and God has forgiven Shawn. God has forgiven me, and I have forgiven myself.'* The more you do this when these negative feelings arise, the more they will weaken and submit to your decision of forgiveness because when you speak against those negative feelings, you're making sure that those feelings hear the truth, which is that you forgave him. You will not fall to the feelings and lies that are coming from your unrenewed mind.

"Listen to me, Tom. It's as simple as this: You'll either believe you forgave Shawn, or you'll believe your feelings. If you truly forgave him, then stand on your decision. That way, you're forcing those old feelings to submit to the decision that you forgave him. I believe you forgave him. I don't care what those old feelings are trying to tell you. You are free from unforgiveness, and I believe you're a man of forgiveness. So, from this day forward, never allow what you feel to decide the choice you made to forgive him. Your feelings are not the governor, you are."

Seconds later Tom said, "Wow! That makes a lot of sense."

Today, Tom says that he no longer has those feelings of unforgiveness against Shawn, and he feels completely free because forgiveness is not a feeling but a decision.

Maybe you're replaying every betrayal, embarrassment, rejection, and disrespect that your mate or spouse put you through in the past. Maybe you're wondering how to forgive them for all the things they did, and all the hurt they caused. Well, what if God treated you the way you're treating them now? Understand this principle: Forgiveness is not for the assailant; forgiveness is always for the victim. In other words, forgiving them helps you; it's not about helping the other person.

We've talked a lot about lies that keep us in bondage. A lie that many people believe is that if you forgive someone who has harmed you, then your forgiveness implies that what they did was okay. The truth is that forgiving them does not make what they did to you okay. The bigger truth is that forgiving them sets you free. There is instantaneous freedom when you choose to forgive. You don't want to remain in bondage to another person who's gone from your life because you refused to forgive them. Your refusal to forgive them will allow them to have control over you—even though you're no longer with them.

Forgiveness is not a mental issue, but a spiritual issue. You cannot medicate a spiritual defect with a worldly mindset. Stop trying to fight a spiritual war by using worldly weapons. You may never understand how and why you must forgive a person to be free; neither do you have to understand why you must obey God and let go of the offense.

Consider this: The choice to forgive or not to forgive happens in your heart, not in your head. When a person has a heart issue and is full of unforgiveness, they refuse to let go of the offense because of their pride. Pride will make them think they're too big to let anything go. That negative pride will cause them to hold onto unforgiveness, thereby making it impossible to forgive the offender. Therefore, they will remain offended and live in bitterness, trapped in pride.

When you choose to forgive an ungodly soul tie for the hurt it caused you, you are killing the negative pride in your heart, and you are regaining ownership of your life. You're making the offender powerless to have any control over your life. Your heart becomes free and clear to develop faith, compassion, mercy, and love, so you can prepare for someone new. Why even consider taking old bitterness into a brand-new, godly relationship? It wouldn't be fair to the next person to get a damaged version of you. You hurt yourself when you justify your right to hold onto unforgiveness.

Someone who is having a head struggle with unforgiveness may have a sincere desire to let it go. Their only problem is that they don't know how to forgive the person who hurt them. As simple as this may sound, all they have to say is, *"I'm releasing the offender. It's over; I'm letting the offense go."* The difference between a heart struggle and a head struggle is desire.

The enemy is the only one who can deceive you into believing that you haven't forgiven, or that you can't forgive. If you accept his lies, then please stop making excuses right now. If you don't want to forgive this person, then be honest and admit that, but don't keep telling yourself lies, because all that's doing is keeping you knitted and attached to an ungodly soul tie. Remember, if you discover the lie and accept the truth, then the lie must die. Plus, the truth will untangle the lie, so you can live free.

Feelings tend to follow the facts. So, the feelings that come with forgiveness may take a little time to settle within you, but as we've learned, each of us is responsible for dealing with our feelings.

Here are four steps to kill the old feelings and develop new feelings:

1. **Make a conscious decision that you will forgive the offender.** Stand on your decision despite what you're feeling.
2. **Stop talking about when, where, how, and why someone hurt you.** The more you feed the past, the longer those past feelings will remain alive. If you starve the past, then those past feelings will die.
3. **When you think about an ungodly soul tie, talk about how much God loves the other person and talk about God's desire to save them.** The will of God is for everyone to be saved even though everyone won't be saved. Therefore, concentrate on His desires for them, instead of focusing on the pain they caused you.
4. **Pray for the other person, as you pray for yourself.** Pray that God will change them and pray that God will keep changing you. If you do this, then every time you forgive, the effects of the ungodly soul tie will die.

CHAPTER 16
OUTGROW IT

As we come down the home stretch, I hope you are feeling your soul tie loosening, even if all the pain hasn't totally left. A piercing may linger, and you're wondering how long it will last. Allow me to expose another lie that may be the final element that is keeping you tied.

Maybe you grew up hearing that time heals all wounds. Honestly, I used to believe it—until I found myself still hurting over things that took place 25+ years ago. I'll never forget the day I was laying on my bed in prison, meditating on all the trauma I had endured in the past. I had changed my life, but I was still hurting. I had cleaned up my language, but I was still hurting. I had cut off all my old friends and distanced myself from anyone who wasn't traveling in the same direction as I was, but the truth was that I continued to hurt.

Unable to figure out why I was still hurting, I told myself that time heals all wounds, hoping I'd feel better. It wasn't two seconds later when I heard a still small voice: *Time doesn't heal all wounds; growth does.*

As I meditated on those words, the voice continued, *"If time heals all wounds, then why do people go to their graves still hurting from the neglect, rejection, or betrayal that took place 40 or 50 years before they died?"*

Instantly I replied. "You're right!" I knew a few family members who went to their graves believing that time heals all wounds and yet they died wounded.

I cannot let you continue to believe a lie that could keep you tied. If you believe that time heals all wounds, you may force yourself to needlessly accept pain from the past. Let's explore this lie and find the truth.

Thinking that time will eventually heal the wound causes you to neglect your responsibility to outgrow what happened to you. It's not your fault that the person you loved betrayed you, abused you, rejected you, disrespected you, or abandoned you. Yet, it is still your responsibility to apply the necessary medicine to heal your broken heart, and this healing medicine is called "growth." If your healing does not happen instantly, then it's God's way of telling you that He wants you to outgrow the hurt progressively.

Please plant this principle into your heart: You don't have a broken heart problem; rather, you may have an inconsistent growth problem. The heart can't stay broken if you're committed to consistently growing. Therefore, by any means necessary, divorce the ungodly or unhealthy soul tie spiritually, mentally, financially, and physically by saying "I do" to personal growth, mental growth, emotional growth, financial growth, and spiritual growth. Every day you neglect growth, you hinder your healing and wholeness, which you will need for your new life in the future.

A lot of people who are dealing with heartbreak focus on healing, but few of them focus on growing. Often, when I coach a person who is dealing with heartbreak, their #1 confession is, "Pastor, I just want to get healed." What they don't realize is that healing comes with growth.

For example, let's hypothetically say, that you got into a physical altercation with your mate or spouse. During the fight, they pulled out a razor blade and cut your arm. The cut was deep and long, so you had to get several stitches. You nursed the wound for a few weeks and then returned to the doctor to remove the stitches. By then, healing was right on schedule. Six months later, your skin had returned to normal. Though you continued to get better physically, every time you looked at the scar, you became furious. Even though the pain was gone, you were still wounded emotionally. You healed but you didn't grow.

After reading and gaining the truth, wisdom, knowledge, and revelation I have given you, none of it will matter unless your focus is 100% on growth. Let's create a daily ritual you can implement to outgrow where and who you are. Sometimes the only way the pain will leave is if you choose to outgrow it.

When it feels like the soul tie has you, I want to show you how to outgrow it. Don't forget that growth is not a one-time event but an ongoing consistent lifestyle. You cannot connect to growth whenever you feel like it; rather, you must stay committed to growth even when you don't have an appetite for it. You can't date growth; you must be fully married to it.

The first hour of your day is the most critical because it can set the tone for the next 23 hours. As soon as you get out of bed, connect with God the Holy Spirit. Jesus said, *"Seek ye first the Kingdom of God, and His righteousness, and all these things shall be added unto you"* (Matthew 6:33). When we put God first on our daily schedule, we make Him our Source. Plus, we position ourselves to receive joy, peace, strength, godly assurance, wholeness, freedom, truth, and love.

Therefore, as soon as you are up in the morning, say the prayer to renounce and break the soul tie. Nothing is wrong with repeating the prayer daily. I want you to say it and memorize it so you will receive a conviction to become one with it.

Next, start thanking God and releasing gratitude for everything he has done and everything he will continue to do for and through you. Thanksgiving and gratitude are spiritual tools that destroy entitlement, pride, arrogance, and depression. Thanksgiving and gratitude will not allow you to stay stuck in your thoughts about what God has not done. Instead, they position you to receive what God is about to do in your life.

As you begin your day with prayer, thanksgiving, and gratitude, you are focusing on how big your God is instead of how big the pain or the problem is.

LIFE-GIVING CONFESSIONS

After prayer, say one of the following three confessions over your life. If you don't speak life over yourself, you can't expect it to come from anyone else. There is life, joy, peace, power, happiness, and direction in the words you speak over yourself.

Right now, open your mouth and repeat this aloud with excitement over yourself:

EVERY SINGLE DAY, IN EVERY SINGLE WAY, I'M GROWING MORE PROSPEROUS; I'M GROWING MORE SUCCESSFUL, AND I'M GROWING MORE VICTORIOUS. I AM MADE FOR PEACE. I AM MADE FOR STRONG

HEALTH, AND I AM MADE FOR GREATNESS. I'M EXPERIENCING THEM IN DIFFERENT DEGREES IN EVERY AREA OF MY LIFE RIGHT NOW. THE FAVOR OF GOD IS UPON ME! THE FAVOR OF GOD IS WITH ME, AND THE FAVOR OF GOD IS WITHIN ME! I HAVE FAVOR WITH GOD, AND I HAVE FAVOR WITH MAN! MY FAVOR IS FOR KINGDOM INFLUENCE, AND MY FAVOR IS FOR KINGDOM IMPACT! I WILL REPRESENT THE KINGDOM OF GOD IN EXCELLENCE AND INTEGRITY, IN EVERY DIMENSION OF MY LIFE! LORD, I THANK YOU FOR WISDOM BECAUSE YOU SAID THAT IF ANY MAN LACK WISDOM, THEN LET THEM ASK OF GOD, WHO GIVES TO ALL MEN FREELY AND WITHOUT PARTIALITY. LORD, I THANK YOU FOR THE WISDOM TO UNTIE THIS UNGODLY SOUL TIE. LORD, I THANK YOU FOR THE WISDOM TO OUTGROW THIS UNGODLY SOUL TIE. LORD, I THANK YOU FOR GIVING ME A VISION THAT WILL PULL ME AWAY FROM WHERE I AM AND PUSH ME TOWARD WHERE YOU WANT ME TO BE. I SURRENDER MY LIFE TO YOUR VISION. I WILL FOLLOW THE LIFE YOU HAVE FOR ME, AND I WILL BE THE PERSON THAT YOU CREATED ME TO BE. I AM NOT POWERLESS. I AM POWERFUL! I AM NOT CONQUERED. I AM MORE THAN A CONQUEROR! I AM NOT A LOSER. I AM A WINNER! I AM NOT WEAK. IN THE NAME OF JESUS, I AM STRONG!

AMEN.

External encouragement from others is good, but internal encouragement from yourself is life changing. On days when you don't "feel like it," you are still the only one who is responsible to speak life into yourself.

Open your mouth and speak it with enthusiasm:

I AM LOVED BY GOD! I AM ACCEPTED BY GOD! I AM AFFIRMED BY GOD, AND I AM APPROVED BY GOD! GOD HAS FORGIVEN ME; THEREFORE, I WILL FORGIVE MYSELF. FROM THIS DAY FORWARD, I RENOUNCE LOW SELF-ESTEEM! I RENOUNCE LOW SELF-VALUE! I RENOUNCE LOW SELF-CONFIDENCE, AND I RENOUNCE LOW SELF-

RESPECT! THE PAST IS BEHIND ME, AND MY FUTURE IS BEFORE ME! GOD WILL WITHHOLD NO GOOD THINGS FROM ME! ON THIS DAY, I EXPECT NEW OPPORTUNITIES, NEW BREAKTHROUGHS, NEW LEVELS OF FAVOR WITH NEW FRIENDS, NEW RELATIONSHIPS, AND NEW ADVENTURES! I WAS CREATED FOR A SPECIFIC ASSIGNMENT: TO ADD VALUE TO THE HUMAN RACE. I AM THE SOLUTION! I AM THE PRIZE! I AM THE REWARD, AND I AM THE ANSWER TO THE QUESTION OF CONFUSION. I MIGHT NOT BE FOR EVERYBODY, BUT I'M THOROUGHLY CONVINCED, AND I'M FULLY PERSUADED, THAT I AM FOR SOMEBODY. I'M GETTING MY LIFE TOGETHER, SO I CAN MAKE THIS WORLD BETTER! MY CHILDREN NEED ME! MY FAMILY NEEDS ME! MY FRIENDS NEED ME! OTHER PEOPLE NEED ME, AND STRANGERS NEED ME TO BECOME THE NEW ME, BUT MORE IMPORTANTLY, I NEED TO GROW INTO THE NEXT DIMENSION, TO WHO GOD IS CALLING ME TO BE! I WILL GROW! I WILL FLOW, AND I WILL GLOW, ALL FOR THE GLORY OF GOD!

AMEN!

Know and believe that your words will create your new world. When things get tight, you must speak life over your own life.

Open your mouth, believe what you are saying, and speak aloud:

MY PURPOSE IS SPECIAL! MY TALENTS ARE SPECIAL, AND MY GIFTS ARE SPECIAL! FOR ME TO EXPERIENCE MY SPECIALNESS, I MUST REMAIN CONNECTED TO A THRIVING COMMUNITY! I CANNOT STAY CONNECTED TO THE UNFAITHFUL! I CANNOT STAY CONNECTED TO THE UNEXCITED! I CANNOT STAY CONNECTED TO THE UNFOCUSED, AND I CANNOT STAY CONNECTED TO THE UNDECIDED, BECAUSE WHAT'S WITHIN THEM WILL EVENTUALLY GET INSIDE ME, AND GOD'S EXPECTATION OF ME IS TO CULTIVATE MATURITY, CONSISTENCY, AND FREEDOM IN EVERY AREA OF MY LIFE. MY EYES ARE FIXED, AND MY MIND IS FOCUSED ON OUTGROWING HURT, LONELINESS, FEAR, AND

THE PAST! WHAT'S BEHIND ME IS DEAD, BUT WHAT'S BEFORE ME IS ALIVE. I MUST BOUNCE BACK! I HAVE TO BOUNCE BACK! I GOTTA BOUNCE BACK, AND I WILL BOUNCE BACK. NOTHING WILL STOP ME! NOTHING WILL HOLD ME, AND NOTHING WILL HINDER ME FROM APPREHENDING MY NEW LIFE THAT GOD HAS PLACED IN FRONT OF ME! I'M EXCITED TO EXPERIENCE THE NEW! I AM READY TO EMBRACE THE NEW, AND IT'S MY TIME TO BECOME NEW!

IN JESUS' NAME,

AMEN.

These confessions will work for you if you believe what you were saying. You must keep repeating these confessions until they become a part of your very being. They cannot be only words on paper, but they must be the life-giving tools you use to help fix your emotions. It's possible only if you believe. If it worked for me and many others, I know it will work for you if you use it. I'll say it again, one of the most powerful verses in the Bible is *"All things are possible to him that believeth"* (Mark 9:23). One of the most powerful weapons in our arsenal is our belief system.

The Bible says, *"Death and life are in the power of the tongue, and they that love it shall eat the fruit thereof"* (Proverbs 18:21). In other words, if life is to flow in you, then life must come out of your mouth. Likewise, if fear or death is to flow in you, then fear or death will come out of your mouth. The enemy knows the power of this principle, which is why he tries to influence you to speak death. Speaking negative words gives depression, despair, and defeat the right to remain present in your life.

Anytime God starts changing you, the first place He begins is in your mouth, because the law of faith says that before you possess a thing, you must first confess a thing. Therefore, nothing will come into your life until you say it aloud. That is why these confessions are so powerful, as you are severing a soul tie.

When I was struggling to get free from a heartbreak and an ungodly soul tie while in prison, I used to say this confession daily:

I AM THE BODY OF CHRIST! THE ENEMY HAS NO POWER OVER ME! I OVERCOME EVIL WITH GOOD BECAUSE THE GREATER ONE DWELLS WITHIN ME! GREATER IS HE THAT IS WITHIN ME THAN HE THAT IS IN THE WORLD. IN MY PATHWAY THERE IS LIFE, AND THERE IS NO DEATH. MY FUTURE IS SOLIDIFIED! MY PAST IS CRUCIFIED! AND GOD WILL BE GLORIFIED IN EVERY DIMENSION OF MY LIFE! MY WIFE IS A WOMAN OF GOD WHO IS BEAUTIFUL ON THE OUTSIDE AND BEAUTIFUL ON THE INSIDE. SHE'S BEAUTIFUL IN HER EXTERNAL LOOKS! SHE'S BEAUTIFUL IN HER FAMILY LIFE! SHE'S BEAUTIFUL IN HER FINANCES! AND SHE'S BEAUTIFUL IN HER FAITH! SHE AND I EPITOMIZE WHAT A KINGDOM MARRIAGE LOOKS LIKE! ON THIS DAY, I AM PREPARING FOR HER! AND SHE IS PREPARING FOR ME! OUR MARRIAGE IS FROM HEAVEN! AND GOD HAS ORDAINED IT TO DESTROY THE WORKS OF THE ENEMY!

Today I am living the fruits of every confession I released out of my mouth back in 2008, when I started saying those confessions. If God's Spirit lives in you, you are designed to create life in the same way God the Father created life when he spoke the world into existence. If he spoke the world into existence, then you and I can speak our worlds into existence. Therefore, don't take your words lightly.

After you speak life over your life, the next step is to develop a time of devotion. In this time, make it a priority to read the Word of God and write down the godly principles you discover. The Word of God is your life-giving source for anything that's malfunctioning in your life. As a child of God, the Word of God is the only authority in your life. Therefore, you must understand it and not make any excuses not to develop a relationship with the Word of God. It's hard to have a relationship with God if you don't have a relationship with His Word.

Jesus said, *"Man shall not live by bread alone, but by every word that proceedeth out of the mouth of God"* (Matthew 4:4). Your body lives by physical bread, but your spirit lives by spiritual bread, the Word of God. God's Word not only feeds your spirit but also renews, realigns, and reconstructs your soul if you accept it and believe it. Once you delete the lies that keep you bound to the soul tie out of your mind, you must fill your mind with the principles of God's Word so that you grow spiritually and mentally. Your mind cannot think different thoughts if it isn't receiving different principles.

If you don't replace the old way of thinking with a new way of thinking, you will end up choosing the same person with a different face. Though you were freed from the old person, you keep the same old mind.

The following is a list of books that I recommend to cultivate a new way of thinking about every area of your life:

- *The Battlefield of the Mind* by Joyce Meyers
- *Your Best Life Now* by Joel Osteen
- *8 Steps to Create the Life You Want* by Creflo Dollar
- *Single, Married, Separated and Life after Divorce* by Dr. Myles Munroe
- *The Spirit of Leadership* by Dr. Myles Munroe
- *The Burden of Freedom* by Dr. Myles Munroe

- *The Supernatural Power of a Transformed Mind* by Bill Johnson
- *Experiencing the Father's Embrace* by Jack Frost
- *The Bait of Satan* by John Bevere
- *Rich Dad Poor Dad* by Robert Kiyosaki
- Switch On Your Brain by Dr. Caroline Leaf

Anytime you develop an obsession for personal growth, you will magnify maturity by reading material that will lead you to where God wants you to be. Reading and studying books will help you develop a better understanding of the Word of God.

SIX WAYS TO KNOW WHEN YOUR MIND HAS BECOME NEW

Accept the truth of this conviction: God wants you to become a better version of yourself. This takes place when you do the work to renew your mind daily. Let's explore six ways of knowing that your mind is being renewed.

1. **You start seeing situations and circumstances from a Heavenly perspective, and not just a human perspective.** For example, since the heartbreak, separation, or divorce was so excruciating, you and your inner circle have always believed that there is no way you could forgive your spouse, move forward, and one day have a great partnership in co-parenting. But since you started valuing spiritual growth and renewing your mind, now you can see exactly how the two of you can work together to make the kids' lives better. You now understand how to see life from heaven's viewpoint, your new place of healing and forgiveness, instead of being trapped inside of a human

perspective, always seeing things or situations from the lenses of negative feelings, to make selfish decisions.

2. **You gain confidence in your God-given authority.** You understand clearly that you are in full control of your thoughts. You start by living from this truth: *"Just because it came into my mind doesn't mean I have to give it attention."* When you have control of your mind, you can take authority over every thought that tries to defeat you. You do not have authority over anything that you've transferred your authority to. For example, you can't have authority over your mind if you've allowed your mind to obsess over any thought. Instead, you must decide which thoughts you will feed your mind. If a thought comes, and it's trying to make you sad, then immediately change the thought! Once you identify the wrong thought, all you must do is choose to think something different. You will break the thought pattern by shifting your attention. Your authority rests on the choices you make.

3. **You refuse to walk in fear.** No longer will you live according to the fearful lie that you'll never find true love after this, or you're too old to be by yourself, so you should just settle for the unpleasant situation. You accept lies like these because you are afraid of an unknown future, but if you renew your mind to God's truth (See: Psalms 37:4), then you will force fear out of your life by making godly decisions and walking in faith. Anytime you feel fear, make your confessions and attack the fear with a decision that flies in the face of what you are afraid of.

4. **You refuse to accept defeat or depression.** Usually, these two nasty and negative emotions come from loneliness. When you've been separated or

disconnected from someone whom you've become one with, it's normal to want to see them and reconnect. The danger of falling victim to loneliness is that eventually you will accept depression and defeat. However, when you renew your mind, you'll know that you may feel weak, but you won't allow that weakness to remain because you'll be in control of your feelings. You'll know that you're not a victim, but a victor. God's Word says, *"God, which always causeth us to triumph in Christ"* (2 Corinthians 2:14). Your new mind will not allow you to stay in defeat or depression. You will know the difference between what you feel and who you are.

5. **You refuse to settle.** When starting over, it's natural to feel inadequate and unloved because the one whom you expected to spend a lifetime with left. Therefore, it takes time to outgrow what they did to hurt you, as well as what they think, say, feel, and/or believe about you. What they think about you can't be why you feel inadequate about yourself. When you renew your mind, what they think, feel, and/or believe about you is nothing of importance to you. You will know that you are worthy of being a lifetime partner to someone who will honor and appreciate you. A new mind will not allow you to settle for what is; rather, it will force you to create what can be. A new mind will not allow you to choose based on where you are but on where you are going.

6. **You refuse to accept dysfunction.** A dysfunctional relationship is toxic, unhealthy, and full of chaos. If you've been in a toxic relationship for a substantial amount of time, it may have become part of the way you do life. You feel like your mate doesn't love you if

you two are not debating, disagreeing, fussing, or fighting. Therefore, dysfunction has become normal to you.

As soon as you start renewing your mind, the spirit of peace comes into your mind and forces chaos and confusion out of your mind. God's principles organize your thoughts and create structure in your mind. Your life resembles stability when your mind is growing past where you are today. Not only can you renew your mind by reading books, but you can achieve this through fruitful dialogue and watching teachings and sermons.

Transforming Faith Christian Center has a plethora of teachings on YouTube. (Please like, comment, subscribe, and share the content.) Take notes and gather principles while you're watching and listening to the messages. Every principle you get, identify where it applies to your life, accept it, and meditate on it until it comes to life within you.

When you start your day off this way, you are resetting and reestablishing your mind to outgrow every hurt, pain, and unhealthy feeling. Throughout the rest of the day, be intentional about the conversations you entertain. If they're not producing spiritual, financial, personal, social, familial, educational, or emotional growth, then refuse to be a part of them. You're in a season of discipline right now. Therefore, if it's not adding value to you, then it's subtracting value from you.

Next, find an accountability partner to walk this journey with you. It's common to connect with people who are going through the same thing as you, but I suggest that you find someone who's already successfully been through the process. Don't connect with anyone whose bitterness is leaking from them. Find someone whom you respect, who demonstrates the fruit of growth, and who gives you the truth with love when you're feeling vulnerable.

Create a daily habit of exercising. You will be surprised at how you'll feel mentally, spiritually, and emotionally. You'll release known and unknown stress that's building up within you. Eating healthy meals is important also. Many people develop eating disorders when they're severing the soul tie. During your free time, work on your vision or do something fun. An idle mind can produce a suspicious mind. The goal is to create healthy habits that will promote daily growth.

When you stay consistent and persistent in growing to become someone new, you will outgrow every hurt or pain you've been through. The steps in this chapter have taught you how to rebuild a new you. Guess what? You haven't seen the best version of yourself until you've outgrown everything that you are used to.

It's time for someone new! Your kids need to see the new you. If they hurt you while they were with you, don't let them continue to hurt you now that they are gone. The new you will not respond to old mistakes, old memories, or old pains. If you're willing to be consistent in this daily regimen, at the appointed time you'll meet someone who's on the same growth journey as you are. God is getting ready to blow your mind!

Remember to sever the soul tie by developing one new growth habit at a time. When it feels like you can't break loose from an ungodly soul tie, then you can always outgrow the ungodly soul tie. That's exactly what I did. I must remind you that it will cost you everything old. If anyone from your old life wants to be a part of your new life, then they must grow with you. If they don't want to do that, then let them go.

It takes consistent discipline and daily sacrifice to grow. It's possible if you believe. If you believe, I'll see you on the other side of brokenness—the place called wholeness. You have the secrets, now it's time for you to untangle the ungodly and unhealthy soul ties and live the wonderful life God designed for you.

We discussed heavy soul ties, moderate soul ties, and light soul ties. What if I told you there is a place of freedom where you can grow into having no unhealthy soul ties. There is a place in growth where you will one day look back at your old self and feel moments of relief, embarrassment (for your old mindset), and at some point you will even laugh at how immature you used to be. This is healthy growth because you are recognizing how far you've come. You'll eventually be in the position to help someone overcome a soul tie. This pain is only for a season. I promise your best days are ahead. Finish the race. Complete the work and get the job done.

Acknowledgments

I want to acknowledge my wife Mrs. Tiffaney Edwards. You're my rib and my rock! Life started showing me a new meaning of what love is, on the day I became one with you. Your love for me is consistently accelerating every fiber of my being. Thank you for pushing me. Thank you for being patient with me and thank you for loving me, not what I can do for you. I truly believe Heaven has new levels of love waiting on us as we continue to grow.

To my Transforming Faith Christian Center Family! Thank you for your support. Thank you for your trust and thank you for being my family. Don't forget, we're just getting started. It's only up from here. The next dimension of freedom awaits us all.

REFERENCES

- Joel Osteen, *Your Best Life Now: 7 Steps to Living at Your Full Potential* (New York: FaithWords, 2014).
- James Strong, *Strong's Expanded Exhaustive Concordance of the Bible* (Nashville: Thomas Nelson, 2009).
- Dr. Spiros Zodhiates, ed., *Hebrew-Greek Key Word Study Bible NIV* (Chattanooga, TN: AMG Publishers, 1996).
- Dr. Myles Munroe, *The Spirit of Leadership: Cultivating the Attributes That Influence Human Action* (New Kensington, PA: Whitaker House, 2005).
- Roswell Hitchcock, *An Interpreting Dictionary of Scripture Proper Names: Showing the Meaning of Nearly All the Names of Persons and Places in the Bible* (New York, 1874).

ABOUT THE AUTHOR

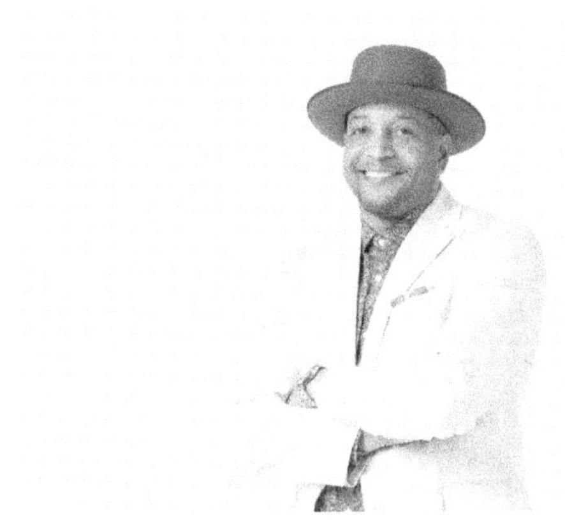

Pastor James Edwards is the Founding Pastor of Transforming Faith Christian Center in Houston, Texas. His challenging life journey was all a part of the process to usher him into the calling God has on his life. James was born in Florence, Alabama. Throughout his childhood, he faced numerous challenges including poverty, abuse, neglect and fatherlessness. He began to equate his self-worth with the unfortunate cards he was dealt in life and made the decision to sell drugs as a teenager.

Eventually, he faced the consequences of his decisions. He was convicted and sentenced to 96 months in federal prison. After 18 months of incarceration, James had a spiritual awakening. He began to question his purpose in life. In that instant, the move of God encompassed his entire being. His quest for Biblical and spiritual knowledge became an obsession. The process of transformation was strenuous, complex and downright painful. James describes it as a crucifixion (dying to himself) and a resurrection (being raised up by God).

Upon release from prison, James was determined to pursue his God-given purpose in life. Within a few years, he became nationally recognized as a motivational speaker, known as *The Most Valuable Motivator*. He relocated to Houston, TX and traveled the United States sharing his life experiences and challenges as a catalyst to transform the lives of others. During this time, he also authored his first book, *"The D.E.A. Will Transform Your Life: A Guide to Mental Transformation"*. Although his gift of speaking allowed him to mix and mingle with some of society's most prominent people, deep down James knew that he had much more than his life story to share. He knew his passion for Christ was the core of his being and the foundation of his life.

Four years into motivational speaking, while on the road to an engagement, James heard the voice of God that said, "Son, people will continue to limit you, label you, and put a lid on your potential until you reveal the 5 different people who are screaming to come out of you. You are a Visionary. You are the Epitome of Transformation. You are the Encourager of Encouragers. You are an Innovator and a Faith Giant." Then God gave James the name for his ministry. From this revelation, Transforming Faith was birthed.

In 2014, James met his wife, Mrs. Tiffaney Edwards. Her purpose intertwined with his vision, and she assisted in the birthing of Transforming Faith Christian Center and continues to uplift and support Pastor James' vision. Together they counsel couples through their marriage ministry, Grace &

Truth. They believe that truth, trust, and transparency gives hope to those who are desperate for transformation and restoration. Pastor James continues to live boldly in truth and freedom. His life is a true testament that God can take our tragedies and turn them into triumphs.

Speaking Engagements
Coaching
Seminars & Conferences
www.PastorJamesTFCC.Church

For speaking engagements, 3 day seminars (soul-ties) conferences, coaching or interviews you can request Pastor James at www.PastorJamesTFCC.Church or email: PastorJ@ TransformingFaith.Church

Follow Pastor James on all of the social media platforms!

http://www.books2read.com/james-d-edwards

facebook.com/100057290604931

instagram.com/pastorjamestfcc

youtube.com/TransformingFaithChristianCenterMedia

tiktok.com/@pastorjamestfcc

twitter.com/PastorJamesTFCC

ABOUT THE PUBLISHER

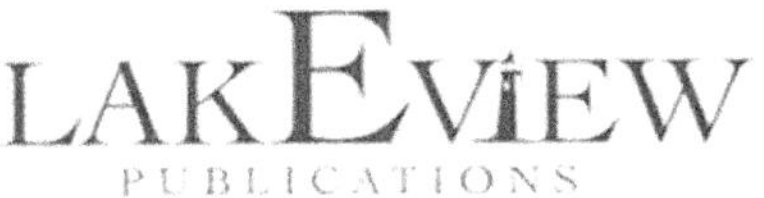

"Everyone has a story to tell, only the courageous will find a way to get it told. Let my team and I help you become courageous!"

Helping people become courageous is something we have been doing sing LakeView Publications was founded in 2018.

With every author we have helped since book one, I am reminded of the day I decided to take the big step of writing my first book. I was quickly overwhelmed with trying to figure out how to bring my dream to life, I just knew that I had a message to share with the world. If you are like I was, You are *NOT* alone! Nearly 100% of our clients started with an idea but had no idea what to do with their idea. That is where my team and I come in. We publish AMAZING books written by AMAZING people who had an idea and took a step in courage to ask the right question. The best way to start, or at least get the next steps is to ask the most important question.

How Do I Get My Book Published?

Finding the right publisher is key. The team at LakeView Publications is driven by our passion to help people tell their stories and in helping them find a way to allow their story to take them to the next level. One of the greatest parts about assisting people in the publishing journey of their story is being able to connect with them and help them find their voice. You reach out to us with the best way to reach you, and we do the rest. It's that easy!

You wrote the book; we do everything else!

When you contact us, we will find out where you are in the process and give you an assessment of what you will need to get you from where you are to where you want to be!

Our team is absolutely magnificent, and they are dedicated to excellence. We offer proofing, editing, layout design, ghostwriting, art illustration, storyboard layout, content coaching, graphic design, and everything else you may need to get your book published and released.

www.LakeviewPublishers.com

facebook.com/LakeviewPublishing

instagram.com/lakeview_publishing

Want to Publish Your Book?

We Can Help!

* Manuscript Editing

* Book Cover

* Book Formatting

*Illustrations

* Publishing through all major retailers
(Amazon, Kobo, B&N, Apple)

* Paperbacks & eBooks

* Blurb Writing

* Audio Books

* Choose Your Own Package

* Author Retains <u>ALL</u> rights

We're here to help!

"Everyone has a story to tell, only the courageous will find a way to get it told. Let my team and I help you become courageous!"

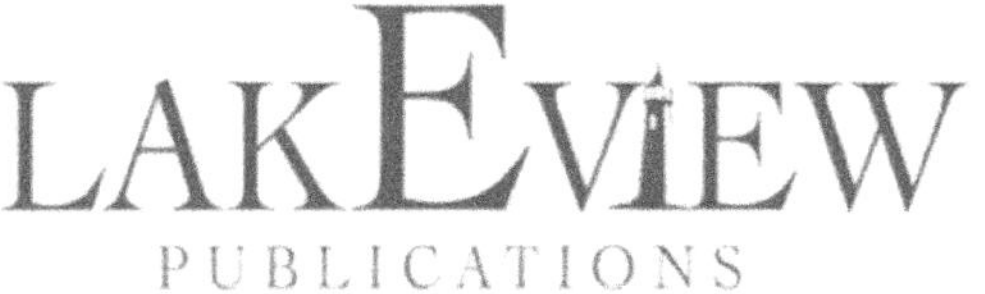

www.LakeviewPublishers.com